Break ICE – The SYSO Way

Basic life support skills and techniques to save lives in case of emergency

Mohan Aakula

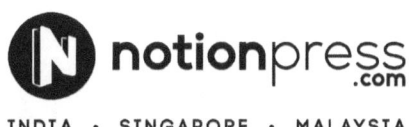

INDIA • SINGAPORE • MALAYSIA

Notion Press

No.8, 3rd Cross Street,
CIT Colony, Mylapore,
Chennai, Tamil Nadu – 600004

First Published by Notion Press 2021
Copyright © Mohan Aakula 2021
All Rights Reserved.

ISBN 978-1-63806-525-8

This book has been published with all efforts taken to make the material error-free after the consent of the author. However, the author and the publisher do not assume and hereby disclaim any liability to any party for any loss, damage, or disruption caused by errors or omissions, whether such errors or omissions result from negligence, accident, or any other cause.

While every effort has been made to avoid any mistake or omission, this publication is being sold on the condition and understanding that neither the author nor the publishers or printers would be liable in any manner to any person by reason of any mistake or omission in this publication or for any action taken or omitted to be taken or advice rendered or accepted on the basis of this work. For any defect in printing or binding the publishers will be liable only to replace the defective copy by another copy of this work then available.

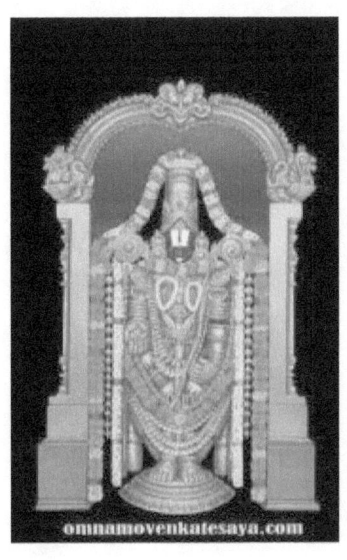

Akalamrutyuharanam, sarvavyadhinivaranam,

Samastha papa kshayakaram, Sri Venkateswara Swamy

padodakampavanamsubham.

The "pujari" in the temple says this while offering "Theertham"

Which means

Let thy be cleared of untimely death and ill health, let all your sins

be cleared at the holy feet of Sri Venkateswara Swamy.

Let's pledge to wipe out untimely deaths.

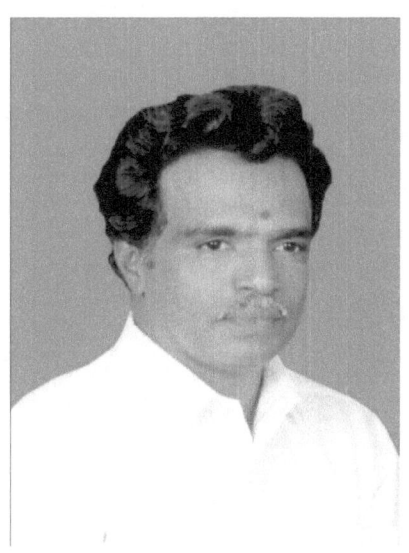

Sri Aakula Subramanyam Garu

DOB: 8-26-1943   **DOD: 10-8-1993**

I dedicate this work to my father Sri Aakula Subramanyam who, in spite of surviving a road accident, passed away due to lack of proper emergency medical care (first-aid). One single life – just one life – it took just that one life lost, to change the course and destination of several lives more fully in the case of his four children – siblings and me.

He had great respect for doctors and had won very many as his friends. He was successful in educating both his daughters as post graduate doctors. Yet that medical care eluded him when he deserved it most. He stood as a living example of SERVICE TO HUMANITY IS THE BEST WORK OF LIFE and continues to. This attempt is one such in that direction.

This book is released on this day the 8th of October 2020 to commemorate the twenty seventh death anniversary of my father.

Contents

Preface	9
Quick Review	13
ICE – Dial 108	19
Emergency Medical ID Card	23
Ice your Cell Phone	26
DIY Survival Kit	29
First-Aid Kit	32
Lifter	34
Automated External Defibrillator	36
Road Safety	39
Fire Safety	43
Basics of Emergency Aid	49
Resuscitation	54
Choking	57
Unconsciousness	60
Heart Attack	63

Importance of CPR	66
Stroke	68
Shock	70
Seizures	72
Head Injuries	75
Asthma	79
Burns	81
Bleeding	85
Diabetes	90
Poisons, Bites and Stings	93
Sprains, Strains and Fractures	97
Facial and Minor Wounds	101
Over Exposure to Heat	105
Frostbite	109
Hypothermia	111
Quicksand	113
Lightning	117
Drowning	122
Snake Bite	125
Blood Donation	133
Eye Donation	136
Organ Donation	139
First Aid Training Institutes	145

Preface

A story goes like this. Three wise and well educated men and a fisherman were sailing in a boat. The three wanted to have fun at the expense of the untutored man. The learned one asked, "Do you know Vedas?" "No, dear sir I don't know" replied the fisherman quietly." A quarter of your life is wasted" quipped the first.

The next one questioned,"Do you know shastras?"" No, my guru no, I don't know" answered the man humbly. "Half your life is gone" retorted the second one. "Atleast, Do you know puranas,?" queried the third one. "No, respected teacher not at all" responded the angler shyly. "Three fourth of your life is fit for nothing" thwarted the third.

Meanwhile the sky grew dark. It was a storm. Waves lashed and the boat was about to capsize. It was the turn of the fisherman to query," oh three of you, the great scholars, Do you know swimming?""No, now…how?" trembled the threesome. "Your entire life seems to be lost" mused the shrimper and swam to safety.

The story goes a little further. The fisherman saved all the three of them one after another by holding their hair and pulling them to the shore. Then he put the water they had swallowed out of their belly by giving them the necessary thrusts, put a fire by gathering the twigs and dried leaves around, for the three to warm up and also found some fruits to nourish them. The world's first first aider was born.

The story goes further a little more. "We grant you a wish" the three cried in unison. The fisherman was unperturbed. "I am satiated to the brim for saving three lives today. If you still wish I command a boon from you, so be it." triumphed the vibrant one

"Learn swimming and savour my feeling" he urged

The moral I have been told was that, having learnt a life saving skill, he saved himself. He was in a position to save others. He was exhausted, no doubt but he was thoroughly satisfied. He had found the meaning and purpose of human life and shared it with others.

Everyone in an emergency situation needs YOU. Visualize how comforting it is to have a dear one with you in such situations. Remember "Do unto others as you would want others to do to you". Replace the words casualty/victim/patient in this book with the word DEAR ONE.

God and god alone can give life. Only some privileged, like the doctors can get most back to life. But anyone like you and me can be an emergency aid responder (EAR) and save lives. "HE could not be everywhere to save lives, so HE made EARs."

Let us dedicate ourselves to eradicate untimely deaths.

Try every means and method, skill and technique to save a life or lives, for you don't get a second chance to do that once it is gone. If it still evades your timely intervention don't put yourself under the risk of losing your life instead as a last resort transfuse the life (lost) into another body through eye/organ donation. Go ahead – Break ice.

The earliest meaning of this phrase, i.e. 'to forge a path for others to follow' refers of course to the breaking of ice to allow the navigation of boats. If we move forward 'breaking the ice' alludes to its original usage, when specialist ice-breaking ships were introduced. These ships, known as ice-breakers, were equipped with strengthened hulls and powerful engines, were employed in the exploration of Polar Regions. Soon after the ships were introduced the term 'ice-breaker' began to be applied to social initiatives which were intended to get strangers acquainted with one another.

"The vanguard never has it easy." Yet be a trend setter, a front runner and a path finder. Be a beacon to show the path and an icon to lead up to. Knowing the problem or reading the situation right is half the solution as the cover design suggests. With the latest technology backing you, put the informative **You** in an **SOS** situation and you have the all pervading **SYSO**.

In any case of emergency, a step by step approach is followed to tackle it. Causes, signs and symptoms, care and management, then the treatment is taken over by the medical staff coming right back to prevention of it all in the first place.

This endeavour explores a step further, the possibilities available the **SYSO** way.

By learning to **s**ave **y**ourself you learn to **s**ave **o**thers. Life is short. In a precarious situation, **s**ave **y**ourself to be in a position to **s**ave **o**thers. Live life to the fullest. Step **y**ourself into the shoes of **o**thers to get their point of view. Live and let live. At the end of life serve **y**ourself well to serve **o**thers. In the military too they follow sacrifice **y**ourself to **s**ave **o**thers. In short the **SYSO** principle. Let it guide you through life and beyond.

The cost of this book is material and therefore immaterial. The purpose of this book is served when some blood donations are effected. The goal of this book is reached when some more eye/organ donations have taken place. The objective of this book is accomplished when this book is able to motivate many more of you to be an emergency resource person.

The aim of this book is achieved when very many more lives are saved. It is then that the value of this is book, is realized and gives immense satisfaction to all involved. Be aware and be ready. You can make a difference, somewhere sometime to somebody, for the rest of their life.

Quick Review

Emergency Management Includes

- Preparedness: Actions taken prior to an emergency or disaster to ensure an effective response.
- Response: Actions taken to respond to an emergency or disaster.
- Recovery: Actions taken to recover from an emergency or disaster.
- Prevention/Mitigation: Actions taken to reduce or eliminate the effects of an emergency or disaster.

Expect the unexpected – an emergency

In a medical emergency, timely response could make all the difference. Here is a checklist of things you should do before, so you are always ready to act quickly.

Get to a hospital in 60 minutes or less

The top three reasons people visit an emergency room (ER) are "heart attack a stroke or an accident" says an ER specialist. In the case of a heart attack or accident, the patient must get to a hospital within 60 minutes. "Go to the nearest big place and not the smallest nursing home close by. Avoid taking an auto, and keep the casualty's spine as still as possible."

Keep your medical history handy

This helps doctors get information such as what the patient has been treated for earlier and what they might be allergic to. To prepare for a situation where you might be the one requiring emergency medical attention, ensure you have a contact person who knows you and your medical history well or has access to your medical files and can bring them to the hospital. It is important to give your primary/family doctor's name and number too.

Know a hospital's emergency services

Most large hospitals have a resident consultant who will be able to diagnose and stabilize you. A good ER doctor will not let you go till your condition is so. That is why it is all the more important to go to a large hospital, as smaller ones tend to keep junior doctors in their emergency rooms.

Keep an ID card with vital details

The biggest mistake people make is not having their basic information in place. A driving license is not enough. Vital details should include your blood group and a contact person in case of emergency. If you are alone, and end up unconscious, this lack of information can leave the hospital in a quandary.

Keep some cash aside

While most hospitals insist that in case of emergency patients are treated without payment, there are family of patients who said they had to pay Rs 15,000/- to Rs 20,000/- before treatment began. A reserve of money at home for a medical emergency might prove helpful. An emergency credit card can also prove to be helpful.

Know what your insurance covers

People should know what insurance they have bought, what they are covered for, what their sub-limits are. The health card from insurance companies has details of the policy and emergency numbers of partner hospitals. Store your insurance policy number and the emergency contact number on your mobile phone too. Call your insurance company within 48 hours of the emergency so that the hospital is notified that the patient is covered by insurance.

Surf the net/telephone directory and make a note of the emergency numbers of all the big hospitals in your town as well as the towns you would be visiting often and in the near future.

A list of emergency numbers, if you are staying at/traveling to the city of Hyderabad.

Ambulance	Medical Services
Apollo Emergency 23548888	Apollo Hospital 23608851
St. John's Ambulance Services 24656785	Care Hospital (Hyderabad) 24735465
Andhra Mahila Sabha: 27617801	Care Hospital (Banjara Hills) 55517777
Pioneer Ambulance:23312145	M N J Cancer Hospital 23318422
Blood Bank	CDR Hospital (Hyderguda) 23221221
Blood Bank Narayanguda 27567892	Gandhi Hospital 27702222
Chiranjeevi Blood Bank 23353114	Govt. ENT Hospital 24740245
MatadinGeol Blood Bank 23226624	Heritage medical center 233799999/23379201
Medwin Blood Bank 23202902/4616	Kamineni Hospitals 24022276
	LV Prasad Eye Institute 23608262
Eye Banks	Mahavir Hospital 23393134
Ramayya International 23548266/67	Mediciti 23237644
Sarojini Devi Eye Bank 23317274	Medinova 23311122/23311133
L V Prasad Eye Bank 23608262	Medwin Hospital 23202902/4000
24 Hours Pharmacy	Niloufer Hospital 23394265
Apollo Pharmacy 23231380	Osmania General Hospital 24600121
Health Pharmacy 23310618	St. Theresa's Hospital 23701013
Medwin Pharmacy 23202902	Nizams Institute of Medical Sciences 23320332/23396552
New City Hospital Pharmacy 55260004	Vijay Marie Hospital 23315055

In Case of Emergency (ICE)

Bring someone with you, or have someone meet you there. Make a list and carry with you at all times: your doctors' names and phone numbers, medications you take, food and drug allergies, a short medical history, phone number of a relative or friend to call in an emergency. Enter your emergency contact into your mobile too. Take time off to pay a visit to the hospital near your home and note the location of the emergency ward. Prepare yourself for the emergency should it warrant itself any moment. To further your cause, talk to the person in charge about how to go about. Make sure your house number is clearly visible from the street. The faster EMRI personnel can find you, the faster they can help you.

14 Reasons to Call Emergency

- Loss of consciousness
- Chest or severe abdominal pain
- Sudden weakness or numbness in face, arm, or leg
- Sudden changes in vision
- Difficulty speaking
- Severe shortness of breath
- Bleeding that doesn't stop after ten minutes of direct pressure
- Any sudden, severe pain
- Major injury, such as a head trauma
- Unexplained confusion or disorientation
- Severe or persistent vomiting or diarrhea
- Coughing or vomiting blood
- A severe or worsening reaction to an insect bite, food, or medication
- Suicidal feelings

Help Yourself: Learn First Aid

"Something as simple as knowing how to apply pressure to stop or slow bleeding can save a life," says MarniBonnin, MD, an ER doctor in Birmingham, Alabama USA.

ICE – Dial 108

108 is a toll free number to call for emergency services in the Indian states of Andhra Pradesh, Gujarat, Uttarakhand, Goa, Rajasthan, Tamil Nadu, Chhattisgarh, Karnataka, Assam, Meghalaya, and Madhya Pradesh. The 108 Emergency Response is a free 24/7 service for providing integrated medical, police and fire emergency services. The emergency telephone number is a special case in the country's telephone number plan. The system is set up so that once a call is made to an emergency telephone number, it must be answered.

Process

When an emergency is reported through 1-0-8, the call taker gathers the needed basic information and dispatches appropriate services. Basic information obtained includes:

- Where the call is placed from (District/Mandal/City/Town/exact location/landmark)
- The type of emergency
- Number of people injured and the condition of the injured
- The caller's name and contact number – for location guidance if required.

Emergency help dispatched through this process is expected to reach the site of the emergency in an average of 18 minutes. Pre-hospital care will be given to patients being transported to the nearest hospital.

The Emergency Response Service should be called:

- To save a life
- To report a crime in progress
- To report a fire
- Anytime an emergency response is required for medical, law enforcement and fire.

In the case of multiple services being needed on a call, the most urgent need is determined, with other services being called in as needed. Emergency dispatchers are trained to control the call in order to provide help in an appropriate manner. The dispatcher may find it necessary to give urgent advice in life-threatening situations and have special training in telling people how to perform first aid or CPR.

International Operation

Many countries' public telephone networks have a single emergency telephone number, sometimes known as the universal emergency telephone number or occasionally the emergency services number, that allows a caller to contact local emergency services for assistance. The emergency telephone number may differ from country to country.

It is typically a three-digit number so that it can be easily remembered and dialed quickly. Some countries have a different emergency number for each of the different emergency services; these often differ only by the last digit. Inside the European Union, 112was introduced as a common emergency call number during the 1990s, and is a well known emergency number in the world today alongside 911 and 999.

In many parts of the world, an emergency service can identify the telephone number that a call has been placed from and can be associated with the caller's address and therefore their location. The latest "enhanced" systems, are able to provide the physical location of mobile phones too.

Emergency Numbers

Mobile phones can be used in countries with different emergency numbers. A traveler visiting a foreign country does not have to know the local emergency numbers. The mobile phone and the SIM card have a pre-programmed list of emergency numbers. When the user tries to set up a call using an emergency number known by a GSM or 3G phone, the network redirects the emergency call to the local emergency desk. Most GSM mobile phones can dial emergency calls even when the phone keyboard is locked, the phone is without a SIM card, or an emergency number is entered instead of the PIN.

Most GSM mobile phones have **112**, **999** and **911** as pre-programmed emergency numbers that are always available. The SIM card issued by the operator can contain additional country-specific emergency numbers that can be used even when roaming abroad. The GSM network can also update the list of well-known emergency numbers when the phone registers to it.

Using an emergency number recognized by a GSM phone like 112 instead of another emergency number may be advantageous, since GSM phones and networks give special priority to emergency calls. A phone dialing an emergency service number not recognized by it may refuse to roam onto another network, leading to trouble if there is no access to the home network. Dialing a known emergency number like 112, forces to call the number with any available network.

On some networks a GSM phone without a SIM card may be used to make emergency calls and most GSM phones accept a larger list of emergency numbers without SIM card, such as *112, 911, 118, 119, 000, 110, 08,* **and** *999.* However, some GSM networks will not accept emergency calls from phones without a SIM card, or even require a SIM card that has credit. For example, Latin American networks typically do not allow emergency calls without a SIM. Also, GSM phones sold in some countries like Singapore do not accept 112 as an emergency number even if they have a SIM card inserted. In the United States, the FCC requires networks to route every mobile-phone and payphone's – 911 call to an emergency service call center, including phones that have never had service, or whose service has lapsed.

Emergency Medical ID Card

The Medical Emergency Card allows medical staff to easily recognize it as your own personal Emergency Medical Identification with instant access to your important medical history and prescription drugs which is very important when a quick diagnosis is vital. Your emergency contacts and physician information are also displayed. An important record, if you are suddenly taken ill or you meet with an accident. It contains your Name, Blood group, A list of your medical conditions, A list of your medications (including herbs and supplements), Name and phone numbers of your doctor, Name and phone numbers of family or close friends, Whether you wear contact lenses etc; It is to be kept right behind your driver's license in your wallet. When the paramedics arrive to help you, they grab a wallet or a purse, so they'll know who you are. They do it consistently. When patients arrive in the emergency room, nurses routinely look for their driver's license to locate next of kin.

In an emergency situation, you may not be able to speak and give vital information to help alert others concerning your health. Medical providers must sometimes treat accident victims without having any basic medical information about the individual or any way to contact someone who could provide crucial information. A medical information card would prove to be invaluable in providing treatment by the attending medics or other medical personnel. A medical identification bracelet or pendant is recommended to alert emergency medical personnel of your medical ID card.

Keeping a personal health record is important even when you're not in an emergency situation. You can present this card to your physician on each visit that list your current medications and other medical information, which will save you time and omission errors, when updating your medical chart.

Therefore create a free emergency medical identification card in a few minutes NOW.

- A medical ID card is one of the least expensive health tools that can save your life. They have saved lives.
- The card can be updated as needed, when medications and health conditions change. Changes can occur frequently.
- The card should be kept with you at all times.
- The card is great when you visit your doctor and he/she asks "what medicines are you taking?" Just show them your card.
- When used with a medical ID bracelet, pendant, etc., the medical ID should include "SEE WALLET" to bring the ER personnel's attention to the card.
- The medical card should be placed right behind your driver's license in your wallet.
- A must for all, particularly the senior citizens.
- Print and Laminate a medical ID card like the sample given below.

Emergency Medical ID Card

Emergency Medical Identification

Sridhar 115, Main St. Charminar Hyderabad 500082.

984802XXX Cell

Blood Type: O –ve

Emergency Contacts:

Monisha-*Wife* 98480XXXXX Cell

Bindu-*Daughter* 98480XXXX Cell

Physicians:

Dr. Naveen, M.D. 98765XXXXX Cell

Dr. Rahul, M.D. 93123XXXXX Cell

Medical Conditions:

Type 1 Diabetic High Blood Pressure Back Pain DVT Right Leg Kidney Stones Medtronic Pacemaker Wear Contact Lens

Medications:

Altace 5 - MG 1xDay Coumadin 5MG-1xDay

Amaryl 1 Tab Loritab 25 MG 1-3xday

Lopressor 50MG-1Xday Altace 2.5MG-1xday

Allergies:

Sulfa Drugs, Keflex, Shellfish Living

Will Organ Donor

-Card Printed: 8/3/2020

Ice your Cell Phone

No one likes to think about the possibility of being seriously injured in an accident, but take a moment to consider what might happen if you're rendered unconscious in an accident or other disaster. How would authorities or emergency personnel notify your loved ones? How would they know your medical history to treat you? By tracing your car's license number or looking at your driver's license, it may not be possible to obtain your home phone number. Moreover, valuable time would be lost searching for information to treat you.

It was from this difficulty in locating family members of accident victims, the ICE idea was born. ICE could save your life. The ICE concept is simple- simply program your cell phone memory with the acronym ICE ("in case of emergency") followed by the names and phone numbers of those whom you would wish to be notified in an emergency. Paramedics, who come in the 108 ambulance, will turn to a victim's cell phone for clues to that person's identity. You can make their job much easier with a simple idea that they are trying to get everyone to adopt: ICE.

For example, "ICE-1 Ramana" as a saved contact entry in your phone would alert emergency response personnel to contact Mr. Ramana at the number listed. You can program as many numbers as you like using ICE-2, ICE-3, etc. so that your emergency contact person's office and/or cell phone numbers are also recorded. Make sure to include your family doctor's contact numbers and the contact numbers of all the doctors you are consulting for all your medical conditions. Also update these from time to time as they are subject to change. It makes sense to insert the relation in brackets for all the ICE contacts since we usually enter and save only the names as we know them and not as how we want paramedics or others to know in case of emergency. Example: ICE 2 Dr.Hari Kumar 944905 XXXXX (family doctor).

You can save them a lot of time and have your loved ones contacted quickly. Programming your cell phone takes only a few minutes to accomplish, yet it may save you and your loved ones hours of anguish in the event of an emergency. Rapid access to your next of kin, who will be able to provide your medical history and any background information needed, can also enhance the success of your emergency treatment.

Paramedics know what ICE means and they look for it immediately. You may consider affixing an ICE sticker on the back of your cell phone NOW to alert emergency personnel to the fact that you have emergency contact information stored in your cell phone's memory. You can also put a sticker on the back of your driver's license or other form of identification so that rescuers will know where to look for emergency contact information.

The campaign is not without its difficulties. Someone besides an emergency responder could call an ICE contact from a lost or stolen cell phone. And many cell phone users use password protection on their phones, and cell phones also might be damaged during a disaster or an accident. That's why people should also keep a card of emergency contacts in their wallet or purse and a medical identification bracelet or necklace pendant to direct attention to where the emergency medical I.D. card is.

In response to this problem many device manufacturers have provided a mechanism to specify some text to be displayed while the mobile is in the locked state. The owner of the phone can specify their

"In Case of Emergency" contact and also a "Lost and Found" contact. For example, BlackBerry mobiles permit the "Owner" information to be set in the Settings -> Options -> Owner menu item. Alternatively, some handsets provide access to a list of ICE contacts directly from the 'locked' screen. Starting with version 2.3 ("Gingerbread"), the Android operating system lets users specify emergency contacts which can be called without knowing the phone password.

There are applications available for some smart phone models that offer the same or more functionality as an ICE phone book entry.

DIY Survival Kit

This application contains how-to articles from wikiHow, the wiki how-to manual. Plus an emergency survival kit stored for offline use. This is a collection of articles to get you through life's most difficult situations. Includes articles on first aid such as CPR, the Heimlich maneuver, treating burns and bleeding. It also contains wilderness life-savers like how to build a fire or find North without a compass. And you never know when you might need some articles like how to escape from a bear or how to survive a riot. Because you never know when you will need this information, the wikiHow Survival Kit is always available - with or without a cellular connection or a Wi-Fi network.

You should get this app and tell your family and friends to put it on their phones too, because you will never know when you will need it.

The two wikiHow iPhone applications are the best way to read wikiHow on your iPhone or iPod touch. The apps enable you to read wikiHow's popular featured article feed, search and browse all of the over 60,000 articles on wikiHow, bookmark articles to store them for later reading, and watch YouTube videos embedded into articles.

In addition, the apps include a wikiHow Survival kit. The wikiHow Survival kit is stored permanently on your phone so that you have it even if you are nowhere near a cell phone or Wi-Fi connection. The wikiHow Survival Kit includes helpful articles on first aid, vehicle problems, wilderness survival, and escaping unexpected emergencies such as riots, and plane crashes.

The wikiHow app is a free download from the iTunes store. Follow these instructions to learn how to install and use the wikiHow iPhone app.

Requirements: Compatible with iPhone, iPod touch, and iPad. Requires iOS 3.0 or later.

Steps

Download the wikiHow Survival Kit app. The wikiHow apps are free applications. Just follow the link to download it from the app store.

Even though the apps are free, you will still need to be signed into a valid iPhone store account to download the app. Your account will not be charged.

Sync your iPhone with iTunes to install the app. Once the sync is completed, you should see a wikiHow icon on the desktop of your iPhone or iPod Touch.

Tap the wikiHow icon to launch the app.

Read the tips. A tips screen with some basic instructions is displayed the first time that you launch the app. Check out the tips, and then press "Start" or "Done" to move on and start using the app.

Explore the main features. The wikiHow app is designed to be intuitive and easy to use. Below are the main features.

The wikiHow Survival kit – The wikiHow survival kit contains articles to help you deal with all kinds of emergencies, from the mundane (jump-starting a car) to the hair-raising (surviving a long fall). These articles are always stored on the phone and are available any time you have your iPhone with you.

Search – Search all of wikiHow. Just type in your query to find all of the wikiHow articles on a given topic. When you're away from the network, you can enable offline search in settings to only return results from articles stored on the phone.

In addition, the apps include a Survival kit. The wikiHow Survival kit is stored permanently on your phone so that you have it even if you are nowhere near a cell phone or Wi-Fi connection. The wikiHow Survival Kit includes helpful articles on first aid, vehicle problems, wilderness survival, and escaping unexpected emergencies such as riots, and plane crashes.

First-Aid Kit

The first-aid kit should contain the following:

1. First-aid manual.
2. Sterile gauze.
3. Adhesive tape.
4. Adhesive bandages in several sizes.
5. Elastic bandage.
6. Antiseptic wipes.
7. Soap.
8. Antibiotic cream. (Triple-antibiotic ointment).
9. Antiseptic solution. (Like hydrogen peroxide).
10. Hydrocortisone cream (1%).
11. Acetaminophen and ibuprofen.
12. Extra prescription medications. (If the family is going on vacation).
13. Tweezers.
14. Sharp scissors.
15. Safety pins.
16. Disposable instant cold packs.

17. Calamine lotion.
18. Alcohol wipes or ethyl alcohol.
19. Thermometer.
20. Plastic gloves. (At least 2 pairs).
21. Flashlight and extra batteries.
22. Mouthpiece for administering CPR. (Can be obtained from local Red Cross).
23. Your list of emergency phone numbers. (Family doctors and close relatives).
24. Blanket. (Stored nearby).

Travel Kit

If you need to fit a mini-kit in your purse or bag, you'll want these essentials:

- Adhesive bandages in different sizes
- Gauze, pads
- Antibiotic ointment
- Antiseptic wipes
- Hand sanitizer
- Adhesive tape

Note: Replace those medications which have been used in case of emergency as early as possible and also check the expiry date of medicines and replace periodically.

Ensure to keep a first aid kit at home and in each of the vehicles the family uses and also at office.

Lifter

In case of emergency, to transport the casualty you can't go get a stretcher. You need a lifter. You need to improvise and make one with the materials available at home or place of work, off hand.

The following are some ways to do that.

1. To improvise a lifter using a blanket and poles, the following steps should be used

    a. Open the Blanket and lay one pole length wise across the center, and then fold the blanket over the pole.

    b. Place the second pole across the center of the folded blanket.

    c. Fold the free edges of the blanket over the second pole and across the pole.

2. To improvise a lifter using shirts or jackets. Button the shirt or jacket and turn it inside out. Leaving the sleeves inside, (more than one shirt or jacket may be required). Then pass the pole through the sleeves.

3. To improvise a Lifter from bed sacks and poles rip open the corners of bed ticks, bags, or sacks, then pass the poles through them.

4. If no poles are available. Roll a Blanket, tarpaulin or similar item from both sides towards the center. Grip the rolls to carry the casualty.

NOTE: If there is any doubt, call the ambulance out.

Automated External Defibrillator

Defibrillation is the definitive treatment for the life-threatening cardiac arrhythmias, ventricular fibrillation and pulseless ventricular tachycardia. Defibrillation consists of delivering a therapeutic dose of electrical energy to the affected heart with a device called a defibrillator. This depolarizes a critical mass of the heart muscle, terminates the arrhythmia, and allows normal sinus rhythm to be reestablished by the body's natural pacemaker, in the sinoatrial node of the heart. Defibrillators can be external, transvenous, or implanted, depending on the type of device used or needed. Some external units, known as automated external defibrillators (AED), automate the diagnosis of treatable rhythms, meaning that lay responders or bystanders are able to use them successfully with little, or in some cases no training at all.

These simple-to-use units are based on computer technology which is designed to analyze the heart rhythm itself, and then advise the user whether a shock is required. They are designed to be used by lay persons, who require little or no training to operate them correctly.

In many areas, emergency services vehicles are likely to carry AED in addition to a manual unit. It is also increasingly common to find AEDs on transport such as commercial airlines and cruise ships. The presence of an AED can be a particularly decisive factor in cardiac patient survival in these scenarios, as professional medical assistance may be hours away.

Automated external defibrillators as public access units are generally found in places including corporate and government offices, community centers etc; In order to make them highly visible, public access AEDs often are brightly colored, and are mounted in protective cases near the entrance of a building. When these protective cases are opened, and the defibrillator removed, some will sound a buzzer to alert nearby staff to their removal but do not necessarily summon emergency services.

How to Operate an Automated External Defibrillator

- AEDs are almost always used on someone that is unconscious. Continue basic CPR until the AED is hooked up and ready.

- Regardless of which brand of AED is used, the only knowledge required to operate it is to press the "ON" button.

- Once the AED is turned on, it actually speaks to you in a computer-generated voice that guides you through the rest of the procedure.

- You will be prompted to place a set of adhesive electrode pads on the victim's bare chest and, if necessary, to plug in the pads' connector to the AED.

- The AED will then begin to automatically analyze the person's ECG rhythm to determine if a shock is required. It is critical that no contact be made with the person while the machine is analyzing the ECG. If the person is touched or disturbed, the ECG may not be accurate.

- If the machine determines that a shock is indicated, it will automatically charge itself and tell you when to press the button that will deliver the shock.

- Once the shock is delivered, or if no shock is deemed necessary, you will be prompted to resume CPR.

Learn CPR for a Loved One.

You don't know when it comes of use to save a life.

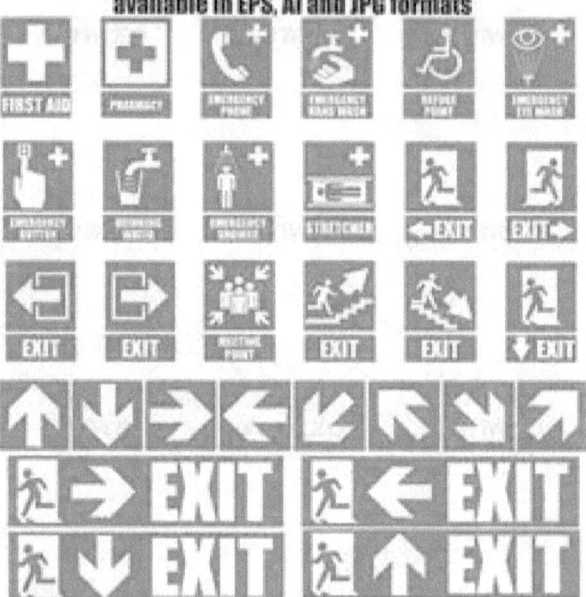

The emergency instructions like which way to get out, where to assemble in case of fire, first aid kit availability, pharmacy, eye wash etc., are all displayed in public places and other areas where people tend to crowd, in the form of vectors.

After all, **"Pictures speak all languages".**

It is important to pay attention and know these signs at leisure, so that they can be followed quickly in case of emergency.

Road Safety

Learning to drive a motor vehicle safely is also a life saving skill for you never know when a medical emergency may call upon you for service or to save yourself. In such situations, you can't keep waiting for a driver or a call taxi to transport the victim. You need to either take out your vehicle or borrow one to reach the casualty/patient to the nearest hospital as soon as possible (ASAP).

Everyone sharing the roads should respect each other's presence and take up the responsibility of the other person as well. Records are there to be broken not rules. Rules are to be followed with pride. Hence follow traffic rules to avoid accidents and thereby emergency situations. After all "Prevention is better than cure".

In order to be safe while walking on roads.

Do's

- The most important road safety tip is to pay attention.
- Always walk on the footpath only. Walk on the extreme right hand side of the road.
- Where footpath is not available so that you can see the traffic coming in the opposite direction.

- Cross only at zebra crossings, traffic signals, subways, foot-over bridges. Where there are no crossings watch the traffic on both sides and cross when it is safe.
- Cross only on a clear green signal.
- Make eye contact with drivers and make sure they can see you.
- Walk between children and the traffic and hold their hands firmly.

Don'ts

- Never cross a road at a corner or curve.
- Do not be impatient, rush or run on the road.
- Avoid walking next to kerb with your back to the traffic.
- Do not read newspapers or look at hoardings while walking on the road.
- Do not greet friends on the road.
- Do not come on to the main road while waiting for a bus. Do not run after, get on or get off a moving bus.
- Do not climb over the barriers or walk between them and the traffic.

In order to be safe while cycling on roads.

Do's

- Wear a cycle helmet.
- Use the cycle lane where ever provided and on the left of the road and traffic, where it is not provided.
- Obey all traffic rules, like the rest of the traffic.
- Look back over your shoulders, give signal and make your intentions clear to the traffic following you.

- Stop before you enter moving traffic from a side lane, parking area or minor road.
- Be careful while passing a stationary car, door may suddenly be opened.

Don'ts

- Never follow any vehicle closely. Maintain safe distance.
- Never ride with one hand on the handle bar except while giving signal.
- Avoid big and busy roads with fast moving traffic.
- Never ride your cycle on a footpath.
- Never try to overtake a fast moving vehicle or which is taking a turn.
- Never ride on the wrong side of the road or cross the road abruptly.
- Never stop suddenly without a signal.

In order to make it safe while driving motor vehicles on roads.

Do's

- Obey all traffic signals, lights and signs.
- Use indicators and signals while changing lanes.
- Always wear safety belts.
- Two wheeler drivers should wear helmets.
- Keep specified speed limits in mind and don't drive faster than the flow of traffic.
- Limit the speed at curves and turns.

- If the vehicle behind you wants to overtake, by all means let it.
- Always carry your Emergency medical ID card and ICE your cell phone.

Don'ts

- Don't drive while under the influence of alcohol or drugs.
- Don't tailgate. Maintain minimum recommended distance.
- Avoid using mobile phones while driving.
- Avoid over loading, over speeding, sudden braking or acceleration.

Be a cautious and courteous driver with due consideration for senior citizens, physically challenged, children, ladies and pedestrians. Start early, drive carefully and reach safely.

Children should be taught the safety code and should not be allowed on to the roads alone until they can understand and follow them properly. Since they learn by example, parents and teachers should always follow the code properly when going out with them.

Note: While on road in a vehicle or otherwise, give way to an ambulance quickly and save lives. Pray and wish for a speedy recovery of the patient whenever you come across an ambulance.

Fire Safety

Do you know what to do if a fire started in your home? Would your kids? Take the time NOW to review fire safety facts and tips to avert a fire accident and also your family will be prepared in the event of a fire emergency at home.

Fire Prevention

The best way to practice fire safety is to make sure a fire doesn't break out in the first place. That means you should always be aware of potential hazards in your home. Start by keeping these tips in mind to avoid an emergency situation.

Studies have shown that many home fires are caused by improper installation of electrical devices. Check all electrical appliances, cords, and outlets

- Are your electrical appliances in good condition, without loose or frayed cords or plugs?
- Are your outlets overloaded with plugs from the TV, computer, printer, video game system, and stereo?
- Does your home contain circuit interrupters/trippers, which prevent electrical shock and fire by shutting off faulty circuits?
- Replace or professionally repair any appliances that spark, smell unusual, or overheat.

- Don't run electrical wires under rugs.

- Make sure lamps and night-lights are not touching bedspreads, drapes, or other fabrics.

- Never place a space heater close to a bed or where a child or pet could accidentally knock it over.

- Keep newspapers, magazines, and fabrics from curtains, clothes, or bedding away from space heaters, radiators, and fireplaces.

Be Careful in the kitchen

Did you know that cooking is the leading cause of home fires in the country? The kitchen is rife with ways for a fire to start: food left unsupervised on a stove or in an oven or microwave (to attend guests or phone calls, chat with friends or watch TV); grease spills; a dish towel too close to the burner; a toaster or toaster oven flare-up; a coffee pot accidentally left on are very dangerous. Always supervise kids while cooking and practice safe cooking habits — like not wearing loose-fitting clothing that could catch fire around the stove.

Beware of Cigarettes

According to the fire department, cigarettes are the No. 1 cause of fire deaths in the country, killing about 1,000 people per year. Most are started when ashes or butts fall into couches and chairs. If you smoke, be especially careful around upholstered furniture, never smoke in bed, and be sure cigarettes are completely put out before you toss them into the trash.

Never let kids Play with Matches and Lighters

Children playing with matches are still the leading cause of fire-related deaths and injuries for kids younger than 5. Always keep matches and lighters out of children's reach. Store, flammable materials such as petrol, kerosene, and flammable cleaning supplies outside your home and away from kids.

Use Candles Safely

As decorative candles become more popular, candle fires are on the rise. If you light candles, keep them out of reach of kids and pets, away from curtains and furniture, and extinguish them before you go to bed. Make sure candles are in sturdy holders made of nonflammable material that won't tip over.

Be aware of Holiday Dangers

Around the holidays, there are even more potential fire hazards to think about. Make sure to switch off the gas connection if you are going out on a holiday. Handle and store fire crackers safely during festive season. Supervise children lighting crackers.

Make sure all smoke alarms are in working order it's a fact — having a smoke alarm in the house cuts your risk of dying in a fire in half. Almost 60% of all fatal residential fires occur in homes that don't have smoke alarms, so this may be the single most important thing you can do to keep your family safe from fires. If your home doesn't have smoke alarms, NOW is the time to install them on every level of your home and in each bedroom. If your smoke alarm uses regular batteries, remember to replace them every year. (Hint: change the batteries when you change the batteries of your clock). Test your smoke alarms monthly, and be sure your kids are familiar with the sound of the alarm.

Keep Fire Extinguishers Handy

Be prepared for any accidents by having fire extinguishers strategically placed around your house — at least one on each floor and in the kitchen (this one should be an all purpose extinguisher, meaning it can be used on grease and electrical fires). Keep them out of reach of children. Fire extinguishers are best used when a fire is contained in a small area, like a wastebasket, and when the fire department has already been called.

The fire department recommends remembering the word PASS to operate an extinguisher:

- Pull the pin. Release the lock with the nozzle pointing away from you.
- Aim low. Point the extinguisher at the base of the fire.
- Squeeze the lever slowly and evenly.
- Sweep the nozzle from side to side.

The best time to learn how to use the fire extinguisher is NOW, before you ever need it. Fire extinguishers have gauges on them indicating when they need to be replaced and should be checked regularly to make sure they're still functional. If you're ever in doubt about whether to use an extinguisher on a fire, don't try it. Instead, leave the house immediately and call the fire department.

Plan Escape Routes

Planned escape routes are a necessity, especially if a fire were to occur during the night. Go through each room in your house and think about the possible exits. You should have in your mind two escape routes from each room, in case one is blocked by fire. Make sure that the windows in every room are easy to open and are not painted over or nailed shut — remember, these may be your only way out in a fire. If you live in an apartment building, make sure any safety bars on windows are removable in an emergency. Be sure to know the locations of the closest stairwells or fire escapes and where they lead.

Teach children the facts about fire.

Teach your kids that fires spread quickly, that most fire-related deaths are not from burns but from smoke inhalation and that dangerous fumes can overcome a person in just a few minutes.

Also to operate the fire extinguisher. Kids should learn to:

- Cover their mouths and noses with a moist towel or an article of clothing to keep out dangerous fumes while evacuating.
- Crawl under the smoke to safety, staying as low to the ground as possible. (smoke always rises)
- Touch any door (not the doorknob) to see if it is hot, and if it is, not to open it (there is fire on the other side) — find another exit.
- Locate the nearest stairway marked "Fire Exit"— kids should know to always avoid elevators during a fire.
- Never stop to take personal belongings or pets or to make a phone call (even to 101) while evacuating.
- Never go back into a burning building once safely outside.
- Stop, drop, and roll to extinguish flames, if an article of clothing you are wearing catches fire.

Practice fire drills at home Fires are frightening and can cause panic. By rehearsing different scenarios, your family will be less likely to waste precious time trying to figure out what to do. Discuss and rehearse the escape routes you've planned for each room of your home. Designate a meeting place outside your house or apartment building that is a safe distance away (a Postbox, a fence, or even a distinctive-looking tree will do) where everyone can be accounted for after they escape.

Then, every so often, test your plan. See if everyone can evacuate your home and gather outside within 3 minutes — the time it can take for an entire house to go up in flames.

Being prepared is the best way to protect your family from a fire. So know the rules of fire prevention, stock your home with fire-safety items, and make sure your kids know what to do in a fire. A few minutes of planning now may save lives in case of a fire emergency.

The neighboring houses would also escape a fire mishap if you followed these preventive measures.

All at home should be taught how to operate a fire extinguisher.

Basics of Emergency Aid

In case of emergency (ICE) preliminary medical care is given to an injured or ill person before medical assistance arrives i.e., Ambulance or the casualty is taken to a Nurse or Doctor.

Assurance

Before the medical care arrives easing of discomfort and anxiety of the casualty is a very important process. Let him/her feel that you are there to be relied upon. Assure the person of your whole hearted help and support. Many people forget that they are treating a 'person', as well as the injury/illness. By combining reassurance with good first aid management, and possibly distracting or diverting the casualty's attention to something else, you will, in most circumstances, actually ease the anxiety and pain levels of the casualty. It would give him the much needed confidence to face the adversity on hand.

By easing anxiety and pain levels you will help to promote recovery of the injured/ill casualty by:

- Decreasing the heart rate.
- This will in turn decrease blood loss.
- Which will in turn slow down the shock process.

Assessment

History – This is the story of the accident/illness which is obtained from the surroundings, the casualty or any bystanders/witnesses that saw the incident.

Signs – This is what you can see, hear or smell, i.e. you can see external bleeding, vomiting, or swelling. You can hear noisy breathing or you can smell alcohol on the breath.

Symptoms – This is how the casualty feels. They can tell you that they feel sick; they have a head ache, abdominal pain or chest pain.

By linking the History, Signs and Symptoms together, you end up with a fair assessment of the injury/illness.

For example:

History – The casualty has had a sudden attack of chest pain which came on all of a sudden and it's been there for 15 minutes.

Signs – The casualty is pale and sweaty.

Symptoms – Central chest pain and the pain is going down the left arm.

Assessment – Possible Heart Attack. Call Helpline Immediately.

Priorities

Life threatening problems are identified and dealt with FIRST. This is done in a strict order of priorities in order to ensure that the most important steps are undertaken in a logical order which will ensure nothing is missed and also prioritize any life-threatening problems.

The systematic approach called **DRABCD** in short is applied to any emergency situation that you go through, from a cut finger to a cardiac arrest. It is also carried in order to ensure the safety of the casualty, any bystanders and you.

D Check for Danger [Hazards/Risks/Safety].

R Responsive? (Unconscious?) If not, CALL Helpline.

A Open Airway. Look for signs of life.

B Give 2 initial Breaths if not breathing normally.

C Give 30 chest Compressions (almost 2 compressions per second) followed by 2 breaths.

D Attach AED as soon as available and follow its prompts.

Continue CPR until qualified personnel arrive or signs of life return

NO SIGNS OF LIFE = Unconscious, Unresponsive, Not breathing normally, Not moving

AED = Automated External Defibrillator

CPR = Cardio – Pulmonary Resuscitation.

D-Eliminate/Minimize the dangers before you approach. Ensure the safety of yourself, any bystanders and the casualty. If it is too dangerous to approach, keep at a safe distance and call the emergency services. Only move the casualty/casualties if absolutely necessary. Ask bystanders to assist you where possible like controlling traffic, phoning for help ASAP (as soon as possible). Use barrier devices where possible like a face shield and gloves.

R-If you have more than one casualty always treat the unconscious ones first. If someone is screaming and shouting and one is on their back quiet, the quiet one has the priority. If they are screaming and shouting, they are breathing.

Use the touch and talk approach. NEVER SHAKE an unconscious casualty. The best way to see if the casualty responds is to use the **'COWS'** method: **C**an you hear me? **O**pen your eyes? **W**hat's your name? **S**queeze my hands.

If the casualty responds, ask their name and carry out the 'History, Signs & Symptoms' assessment principle. If an ambulance is required, call '108' now. If you are in any doubt, call the ambulance out. If the casualty is unconscious, not responding to talk and touch, call '108' now and move onto the airway.

A – The guidelines state 'The casualty should not be routinely rolled onto the side to assess airway and breathing. Assessing the airway of the casualty without turning onto the side (i.e. leaving them on their back or in the position in which they have been found) has the advantages of simplified teaching, taking less time to perform and avoids movement.

The exceptions to this would be in submersion injuries or where the airway is obstructed with fluid (vomit or blood). In this instance the casualty should be promptly rolled onto the side to clear the airway.

Keeping the head in the position you found it, look in the mouth. If any solid or liquid is found, place the casualty onto their side and clear the airway.

If nothing is found in the mouth, leave the casualty on their back and open the airway using the head tilt/chin lift techniques. Place one hand on the casualty's forehead and two fingers under the chin. Tilt the head back and lift chin up opening the airway.

Warning: Once the airway is obstructed, an oxygen deficiency develops in the brain resulting in unconsciousness. Death will follow rapidly if breathing is not promptly restored.

B–Check the casualty's breathing by placing your ear and cheek by their mouth and nose whilst looking at their chest:

- Look for movement of their chest and upper abdomen.
- Listen for normal breathing
- Feel for breath on the side of cheek

Normal breathing is between 12–24 breaths per minute. Assess their breathing for no longer than 10 seconds before deciding whether breathing is normal or not. You are assessing for more than the occasional gasp of air.

If the casualty is breathing normally, place them onto their side if not already done. Call 'Emergency' and assess their airway and breathing every minute. If the casualty is not breathing, not breathing normally or there is any doubt to whether they are breathing normally, call '108' and then carry out 2 rescue breaths.

Ensuring the head is tilted back and the chin lifted up, seal their mouth with yours and blow in for approx. 1 second. Look out the corner of your eye for normal rise of the chest. Take your mouth off theirs and watch the chest fall, take another normal breath and breathe into the casualty again. Check quickly for normal breathing. If the casualty has begun to breathe normally, place them onto their side and assess their airway and breathing until medical aid arrives. If the casualty has not started breathing normally after 2 rescue breaths, carry out chest compressions immediately.

C – Place the heel of one hand on the center of the chest (lower half of the sternum) with your other hand on top. Interlock fingers and pull your fingers off the rib cage. Press down on the chest to a depth of 1/3. Compress the chest 30 times at a rate of 100 compressions per minute. Once you have carried out 30 chest compressions, carry out 2 rescue breaths.

Continue at a ratio of 30:2 until either:

- Professional arrives to relieve you.
- The casualty begins to breathe normally.
- It becomes too dangerous to continue.
- You become too exhausted to continue.
- Another competent first aider takes over from you.
- The casualty begins to vomit.
- A doctor pronounces death.

D-Attach an Automatic External Defibrillator (AED) if available and follow the voice prompts.

Resuscitation

A person who is having difficulty breathing is in respiratory distress. A person who is not breathing is in respiratory arrest. A person in respiratory arrest needs resuscitation. When a person is in respiratory arrest, the heart may still be beating. Without resuscitation, the heart will stop beating soon after breathing stops. In some instances the heart may stop beating first, and then breathing stops immediately. This casualty needs cardio-pulmonary resuscitation (CPR), which combines rescue breathing, with external chest compressions (ECC) to circulate the blood. Properly performed CPR can keep a casualty's vital organs supplied with oxygen-rich blood until ambulance personnel arrive to provide advanced care.

Ratio for adult CPR

30 compressions + 2 Rescue breaths

5 times for every 2 minutes

Remember, any resuscitation is better than no resuscitation at all. If you are unwilling or unable to carry out rescue breaths, then at least carry out chest compression – basic life support. If you don't do anything the casualty will die.

Mouth to Nose Technique

a. Close the casualty's mouth with the hand that is supporting the jaw.

b. Apply the head tile and seal the lips with the thumb.

c. Blow into the casualty's nose.

d. Turn your head to the side, look, listen, feel.

e. Providing resuscitation for a casualty with a possible head, neck or back injury.

If you suspect a casualty has sustained a head, neck or back injury, you should try to minimize movement of the head, neck and spine as much as possible. If your casualty is not breathing resuscitation must still be performed and, if possible, you should use jaw thrust and not head tilt and jaw support.

Reasons for use:

- Rescuer's choice
- Jaw clenched tight
- When resuscitating in deep water
- Major mouth/jaw injuries

Mouth to Mask Technique

The mouth-to-mask avoids mouth-to-mouth contact between the first aider and the casualty. Whenever available, this method should be used as it is more hygienic. Resuscitation should not be delayed whilst waiting for the mask to arrive.

a. Position yourself at the head of the casualty. Ensure a firm seal over both mouth and nose.

b. Maintain head tilt, jaw thrust and breathe into the mask. Remove your mouth from the mask, move your head to the side keeping your eyes on the chest to check for inflation and also allow the casualty to exhale.

c. Can also be delivered from beside casualty. Place mask over mouth & nose and hold in place using pistol grip.

Child (1–8 years)

Head tilt will carry according to the development of the child.

a. Gently breathe air into the child using just enough pressure to make the chest rise.

b. If the breath does not go in, check the airway is open. More head tilt may be needed to open the airway.

c. Use pistol grip to support jaw.

d. Compressions 1/3 of chest using 1 hand.

e. Follow same procedure for resuscitation on adults. (i.e. 2 rescue breaths, 30:2, 5 cycles in 2 minutes).

Warning: The casualty should be continually monitored for development of conditions which may require the performance of necessary basic lifesaving measures such as clearing the airway and mouth to mouth resuscitation.

"If an objects in the body (fails to exit) do not attempt to remove it or probe the wound. Apply a dressing.

Apply a dressing around the object and use additional improvised bulky materials/dressing to build up the area around the object to stabilize the object and prevent further injury."

Casualties with lower jaw [mandible] fractures cannot be laid flat on their backs because facial muscles will relax and may cause an airway obstruction.

Choking

Airway obstruction may be partial or complete and may be present in the conscious or unconscious casualty.

Some causes of Upper Airway Obstruction could be:

- Relaxation of the airway muscles due to unconsciousness
- Inhaled foreign body
- Trauma to the airway
- Anaphylactic reaction
- Partial Obstruction

Signs and Symptoms

With a partial obstruction, some air will be getting past the obstruction into the lungs.

The casualty may present the following signs and symptoms.

- Difficulty breathing
- Wheezing and snoring sounds
- Persistent cough

Care and Management

- Despite evidence of an obstruction, if the casualty is coughing encourage them to cough to try and dispel the obstruction.
- Reassure the casualty and get the history.
- DO NOT carry out back slaps as this may make the situation worse.

Full Obstruction

Signs and Symptoms

- Unable to speak, cough, breathe or cry.
- Blue tinge of the lips.
- The casualty may grip their throat.
- Agitated and distressed.
- Rapid loss of consciousness.

Care and Management

- Call 'Emergency'
- Calm and reassure the casualty
- Administer up to 5 back slaps (these are carried out by using the heel of your hand in an upward movement between the shoulder blades). Check to see if each blow has relieved the obstruction. An infant may be placed in a head downwards position prior to delivering back blows, i.e. across the rescuers lap.
- If back blows are unsuccessful, carry out up to 5 chest thrusts checking after each thrust to see if the obstruction has been relieved.
- If the obstruction is still not relieved, continue alternating between 5 back blows and 5 chest thrusts until either the

ambulance arrives, the obstruction is relieved or the casualty goes unconscious.

- If the casualty goes unconscious, place them into the recovery position and check airway and breathing. If the casualty is not breathing normally, begin CPR.
- Seek Medical advice.
- Apply Heimlich maneuver.

Heimlich Maneuver on an Adult

If the person is sitting or standing, stand behind him or her. Form a fist with one hand and place your fist, thumb side in, just below the person's rib cage in the front. Grab your fist with your other hand. Keeping your arms off the person's rib cage, give four quick inward and upward thrusts. You may have to repeat this several times until the obstructing object is coughed out.

If the person is lying down or unconscious, straddle him or her and place the heel of your hand just above the waistline. Place your other hand on top of this hand. Keeping your elbows straight, give four quick upward thrusts. You may have to repeat this procedure several times until the obstructing object is coughed out.

Note: To perform chest thrusts identify the same compression point as for CPR and give up to 5 chest thrusts. These are similar to chest compressions but sharper and delivered at a slower rate. The infant should be placed in a head downwards supine position across the rescuers thigh. Children and adults may be treated in the sitting or standing position.

Warning: If the casualty is lying on his chest [prone position] cautiously roll the casualty as a unit so that his body does not twist. [Which may further complicate a back, neck or spinal injury].

Do not move casualty to place padding.

Unconsciousness

Unconsciousness is a state of unresponsiveness, where the casualty is unaware of their surroundings and no purposeful response can be obtained.

The brain requires a constant supply of oxygenated blood and glucose to function. Any interruption in this supply will cause loss of consciousness within a few seconds and permanent brain damage in minutes.

Causes

The causes of unconsciousness can be classified into four broad groups:

- Blood circulation problems
- Blood oxygenation problems
- Metabolic problems (diabetes, overdoses)
- Central nervous system problems (Head injury, stroke, tumor, epilepsy)

The best way to remember the common causes of unconsciousness is with the mnemonic FISH SHAPED.

They are Fainting, Imbalance of Heat, Shock, Head Injury – Stroke, Heart Attack, Asphyxia (choking), Poisoning, Epilepsy and Diabetes.

Positioning of the Unconscious Casualty

With an unconscious casualty, care of the airway takes precedence over any injury including the possibility of a spinal injury. All casualties' that are unconscious and breathing normally must be placed into the recovery position to:

- Obtain and maintain a clear airway
- Provide ready access to the airway
- Facilitate drainage and lessen the risk of inhaling foreign material
- Avoid unnecessary bending and twisting of the neck
- Permit continuous observation of the casualty

Please note that a pregnant lady who is unconscious and breathing normally must be, where possible, be placed on their left side. This is to prevent the baby placing pressure on the main vein which will stop de-oxygenated blood coming back into the right side of the heart to be oxygenated. A good way to remember this is "Labour Left".

Fainting

Fainting is a common cause of unconsciousness and may occur when the casualty's heart rate is too slow to maintain sufficient blood pressure for the brain. This is a partial or complete loss of consciousness caused by a relative lack of blood flow to the brain.

Fainting usually occurs because of one of three processes:

- Seizure activity
- Inadequate supply to the brain (Low blood sugar)
- Inadequate oxygen supply to the brain

Signs and Symptoms

Fainting may occur with or without Warning.

- Feeling light headed or dizzy
- The signs of shock, such as pale, cool, moist skin
- Nausea (Feeling Sick)
- Numbness or tingling in the fingers and toes

Care and Management

Usually, fainting resolves itself. When the casualty collapses, normal circulation to the brain resumes. The casualty usually regains consciousness within a minute or two. Fainting does not usually harm the casualty; however injury can occur from falling onto the floor.

- Call Emergency
- RABC
- If the casualty responds, leave them on their back.
- If possible, raise the casualty's leg approx. 20–30cm.
- Loosen any restrictive clothing around the waist and neck.
- If the casualty is unresponsive, unconscious and breathing normally place them into the recovery position, call helpline and monitor their Airway and Breathing until help arrives.
- Shift the casualty to the hospital.

Usually, the casualty who faints will recover with no lasting effects. However, because you may not be able to determine whether the faint is linked to a more serious condition, the casualty should seek/taken for medical attention.

Heart Attack

Heart disease is the biggest cause of death in the world. It is vitally important to get the casualty to hospital if you suspect they are having a heart attack. Early recognition and management is essential and "every minute counts". Dial helpline call ambulance immediately.

Causes

- Smoking
- Stress
- High blood pressure
- Poor diet
- High cholesterol
- Lack of exercise
- Genetics

There are seven causes of heart disease. We can do something about six of these seven, so "Why is heart disease the biggest killer in the world?"

Angina

This is a condition which occurs when the coronary arteries become seriously narrowed by disease and the supply of oxygenated blood to the heart becomes insufficient for the increased oxygen required during an activity.

Signs and Symptoms

- Chest pain is usually associated with exertion or stress
- The pain may radiate to the neck, jaw, shoulder or arms.

  (Usually the left arm)
- Shortness of breath

Care and Management

- History (Do they suffer from heart disease and are they on any prescribed medication for it)
- Rest the casualty, sitting if possible and reassure them
- Assist the casualty to "self-administer" their own medication if they haven't already done so. (If they have self-administered their own medication, do not tell them to take more unless advised to do so by the ambulance operator)
- If the rest and medication does not resolve the problem, then call "Emergency" immediately
- If the casualty becomes unconscious follow the DRABCD principle and resuscitate if necessary.
- Shift the casualty to the hospital as soon as possible.

Heart Attack

This occurs when an artery supplying the heart with oxygen (coronary artery) is blocked. The part of the heart where the blockage is will not receive oxygen and will die. This is termed a heart attack. This is usually sudden onset and the casualty may not have any history of heart disease.

Signs and Symptoms

- Severe central chest pain described as a heaviness or crushing sensation on the chest, radiating to the arms, jaw, shoulders, neck and back
- May occur at rest
- The pain may not be relieved by rest
- Pale, cool and clammy (Cardiogenic shock)
- Breathing difficulty
- Sweating
- Nausea and vomiting
- Dizziness
- May feel terrified and have a feeling of impending death

Care and Management

- ABCD
- Call ambulance immediately.
- Rest and reassure the casualty
- DO NOT allow the casualty to walk about.
- Assist with any prescribed medication.
- Make sure you stay calm.
- Be prepared to carry out resuscitation.
- Seek medical advice.
- Shift the casualty to the hospital as soon as possible.

Importance of CPR

Cardiac Arrest

When a person develops cardiac arrest, the heart stops beating. There is no blood flow and no pulse. With no blood flowing to the brain, the person becomes unresponsive and stops breathing normally.

When you discover a person whom you believe is experiencing a medical emergency, the first thing to do is check for responsiveness. Gently shake the victim and shout, "Are you OK?"

If the person does not respond to your voice or touch, they are unresponsive. If the victim is unresponsive and you are alone, leave the victim and immediately call ambulance. If someone is with you, tell him or her to go call ambulance and then return to help you.

If an AED is available, bring it to the person's side. The moment an AED becomes available press the "on" button IMMEDIATELY. The AED will begin to speak to you. Follow its directions to use the AED. Minimize interruptions in chest compressions before and after each shock. Resume CPR beginning with compressions immediately after each shock.

Chest Compressions

While waiting for help or an AED, begin CPR. Start with chest compressions. Here's how:

- Place the heel of one hand on the center of the chest, right between the nipples. Place the heel of your other hand on top of the first hand and interlace fingers. Lock your elbows and position your shoulders directly above your hands.

- Press down on the chest with enough force to move the breastbone down about 2 inches in adults and children or 1.5 inches for an infant (these guidelines exclude newborns).

- Compress the chest 30 times, at a rate of about 100 times per minute or more. (That's about the same rhythm as the beat of the Bee Gee's song "Staying' Alive").

Airway and Breathing

- If you've been trained in CPR, you can now open the airway by tilting the head back and lifting the chin.

- Pinch closed the nose of the victim. Take a normal breath, cover the victim's mouth with yours to create an airtight seal, and then give two, one-second breaths as you watch for the chest to rise.

- Continue compressions and breaths—30 compressions, two breaths—until help arrives.

Note: This reference is only intended to serve as a guideline for learning about CPR. It is not intended to be a replacement for a formal CPR course. If you are interested in taking a CPR course contact any of the recognized and reputed first aid training institutes in your local area/the Red Cross by phoning your local chapter. Never practice CPR on another person, because bodily damage can occur.

Learn CPR for a loved one.

You don't know when it comes of use to save a life.

Stroke

A stroke occurs when the supply of blood to part of the brain is suddenly disrupted. Oxygenated blood is carried to the brain in arteries. The blood in these arteries may stop moving because of either a clot blocking the artery or a rupture in the blood vessel.

When blood flow to part of the brain is inadequate, the cells in that area will die and the brain can become permanently damaged. Stroke is currently the most common cause of death after heart disease. However, there is good evidence that the outcome can be improved through urgent admission to hospital, therefore the need for early recognition and management is essential.

Signs and Symptoms

The Warning signs of stroke may include one or more of the following:

- Weakness, numbness or paralysis of the face, arms or legs.
- Difficulty communicating (speaking or understanding)
- Difficulty swallowing
- Dizziness, loss of balance or unexpected fall
- Loss of vision, sudden blurred or decreased vision in one or both eyes

- Sudden onset of headache
- Drowsiness

FAST is a simple way of remembering the signs of stroke

Facial weakness – can the person smile? Has their mouth or eye drooped?

Arm Weakness – can the person raise both arms?

Speech difficulty – can the person speak clearly and understand what you say?

Time to act FAST – Seek medical attention immediately. Call emergency helpline.

Care and Management

- Call ambulance and stay with the casualty.
- If the casualty is conscious provide reassurance, make the casualty comfortable and do not give them anything to eat or drink.
- If the casualty is unconscious, follow ABC principle. If they are unconscious and breathing normally, place them into the recovery position and monitor their airway and breathing until medical help arrives.

Shock

Shock is a term used to describe the lack/loss of effective circulation. Shock thus causes failure of the circulatory system to provide adequate oxygen rich blood to all parts of the body. If the vital organs do not receive enough oxygen rich blood, death will occur.

Causes

- Low blood volume due to bleeding, vomiting or diarrhea
- Heart attack or irregular rhythms
- Spinal cord injury
- Severe burns
- Severe sweating and dehydration
- Infections or allergic reactions
- Injury

Signs and Symptoms

- Pale, cool, moist skin
- Rapid breathing
- Rapid and weak pulse

- Confused/disorientated
- Excessive thirst
- Nausea and/or vomiting
- Altered level of consciousness.

Care and Management

- Ensure the area is safe, follow RABCD of first aid
- Stop any obvious bleeding
- Call ambulance
- Rest the casualty comfortably and elevate their legs if other injuries permit you to do so. Do not elevate if legs are fractured, heart attack, head or spinal injuries.
- Keep the casualty warm.
- Care for any other injuries or wounds.
- Monitor airway and breathing and record findings.
- If the casualty becomes unconscious, place in a lateral position.
- Moisten casualty's lips if thirsty but do not give anything to eat or drink.
- Shift the casualty to the hospital as soon as possible.

Seizures

Causes

A seizure may occur for various reasons such as:

- In a person with epilepsy.
- In most conditions effecting the brain (head injury, stroke, meningitis, brain tumor, and lack of oxygen to the brain).
- Poisons and drugs.
- Withdrawal from alcohol or other drugs.
- In children under five years of age due to a sudden rise in temperature (febrile convulsion).

Signs and Symptoms

There are many different types of seizure and the signs and symptoms may vary from person to person. Seizures not resulting in a loss of consciousness require little first aid management other than reassurance and protection from injury.

However, in a major seizure which is commonly termed a "tonic clonic" seizure, good first-aid management is vital. The signs and symptoms are:

- Sudden spasm of the muscles producing rigidity and the casualty will fall down. This is known as the "tonic phase".

- Violent jerking movements of the arms, legs and head may occur. This is known as the "clonic phase".
- Unconsciousness
- Noisy breathing
- Salivation
- Urinary incontinence

Care and Management

- Call Emergency
- Make sure the area is safe and move any objects away so that the casualty will not injure themselves.
- Do not restrain the casualty during the seizure unless it is essential to avoid injury.
- Place the casualty onto their side (recovery position) as soon as possible to open and maintain a clear airway.
- Check the casualty for breathing and if not breathing, resuscitate.
- Allow the casualty to sleep under supervision once the seizure stops.
- Do not attempt to place anything into the casualty's mouth.
- Protect the head from hitting the floor during the seizure by placing something soft underneath their head.
- Seek medical advice immediately.

Febrile Convulsion

This is due to a sudden rise in temperature, usually above 38 degrees Celsius.

Febrile convulsions occur in approximately 3% of children during the first 5 years.

Causes

Febrile convulsions are brought on by a high fever which is usually caused by a viral infection.

Care and Management

- Follow the guidelines for the management of a seizure.
- Following the seizure, leave the child resting on their side.
- Seek medical advice as soon as possible for the treatment of any underlying infection.

When to call an ambulance

- The seizure lasts more than a few minutes
- The casualty has repeated seizures
- The casualty has injured himself
- The casualty is pregnant
- The casualty has diabetes
- The casualty is an infant or child
- It is the casualty's first ever seizure
- The seizure has taken place in water
- The casualty remains unconscious

You are uncertain about the cause of the seizure

Note: If there is any doubt, call the ambulance out.

Head Injuries

Injuries to head are of three types. They are:

- Concussion
- Cerebral compression
- Skull fracture

Concussion

Concussion is a temporary impairment of brain function, usually without permanent damage.

Signs and Symptoms

- Brief period of Unconsciousness
- Blurred vision, Seeing Stars
- Headache, Vomiting
- Dizziness
- Lack of Co-Ordination
- Short Term Memory Loss

Care and Management

- Assess the conscious state.
- If unconscious place them in a lateral position.
- If conscious continue to observe the casualty, noting any change.
- A doctor should rule out the possibility of other associated injuries.

NOTE: Anyone who has been knocked down unconscious playing sports should not play until they have seen a doctor.

Cerebral Compression

This is a condition of increased pressure on the skull that compresses the brain tissue and disrupts brain function.

Causes

- Direct violence to the head
- Skull fracture
- Bleeding/bruising inside the skull
- Tumors
- Infections of the brain (meningitis)

Signs and Symptoms

- Altered conscious state
- Noisy/Irregular breathing
- Weakness on one side of the body
- Unequal pupils
- Flushed/red face
- Aggressive/agitated behaviour

Care and Management

- Call ambulance immediately (even if the casualty is conscious).
- Unconscious casualty – lateral position, observe ABC continually.
- Conscious casualty – instruct the casualty not to move in case of spinal injury.
- Monitor vital signs, and care for other injuries.
- Seek medical advice.
- Shift the casualty to the hospital as soon as possible.

Skull Fracture

A breakage of the skull bone is termed skull fracture.

Signs and Symptoms

- Bruising or lacerations
- Unequal pupils
- Bloodshot or black eyes
- Blood or fluid oozing from the ear or nose
- Altered conscious state

Care and Management

- Call ambulance (even if they are conscious).
- If unconscious – lateral position and observe ABC continually.
- If conscious – support the casualty in a half sitting position and continually monitor ABC.
- If blood or a semi-clear fluid is discharging from an ear, place the casualty in the lateral position to allow the fluid to drain

from the ear. Cover the affected ear but do not plug the ear canal. Monitor and record the vital signs.

- Seek medical advice.
- Shift the casualty to the hospital as soon as possible.

Warning: when the dressing is applied, do not put pressure on the wound or exposed internal parts, because pressure could cause further injury (vomiting, ruptured intestine, and so forth). Therefore the dressing ties (tails) loosely at casualty's, not directly over the dressing.

Asthma

This is a condition where the air passages to the lungs become narrowed by muscle spasm, swelling of the mucous membrane lining the lungs and increased mucous production in the lungs. The airways become narrowed and the casualty will experience difficulty in breathing. Air is trapped in the lungs because the casualty cannot easily breathe out.

Causes (Asthma Triggers)

- Colds and infections
- Exercise
- Inhaled allergens (pollens, moulds, animal dandruff, house dust mites)
- Sudden weather and temperature changes
- Tobacco smoke
- Food additives
- Emotions or stress

Signs and Symptoms

- Shortness of breath
- Unable to finish full sentences

- Dry or moist cough
- Increased heart rate
- Blueness of the lips
- Exhaustion
- Anxious and distressed
- Wheezing

Please note that if the casualty is suffering a severe asthma attack and their wheeze disappears they need hospital treatment immediately. It takes two things to make a wheeze: narrowed airways and airflow. If the attack is very severe and there is scarcely any air moving in and out of the lungs, wheezes may be absent. "IN AN ACUTE ASTHMA ATTACK, SILENCE IS NOT GOLDEN - IT'S DEADLY".

Care and Management

- Sit the casualty upright and give reassurance. Do not leave the casualty alone.
- If the casualty is co-operative, give 4 puffs of a bronchodilator every 4 minutes. A spacer should be used if available.
- If there is no improvement after 4 minutes, call "Emergency".
- If the casualty is unable to take the medication, call "Emergency".
- If the casualty becomes unconscious, DRABCD and resuscitate if necessary.
- Seek medical advice.

Burns

A burn is an injury resulting from heat, chemicals, electricity or radiation. The severity of the burn depends on a number of factors:

- Size of the burn (the amount of area covered)
- Cause of the burn (Chemical, electricity)
- Age (the young and old are more at risk)
- Location (where on the body the burn is. Facial burns could cause airway obstruction)
- Depth (the deeper the burn, the worse it will be)

Classification of Burns

- Superficial (1st degree burn)
- Partial (2nd degree burn)
- Full thickness (3rd degree burn)

A superficial burn is the least severe form of burn and affects the outer layer of the skin known as the epidermis. This type of burn has the appearance of being red, swollen and painful. An example of a superficial burn is perhaps from the steam from a boiling jug or hot iron. The burn is considered to be minor if the area does not cover more than the size of the casualty's palm of their hand.

A partial thickness burn is more severe. With this burn the epidermis and dermis layers of the skin are affected. This burn is considered to be minor if the area involved is no greater than the size of a coin.

A full thickness burn is very severe. All layers of the skin are affected. The burn is black and charred the deeper it is and non-painful in the centre of the burn as the nerve endings have been affected. There is pain associated with this burn and that comes from the outer edges of the burn that will be superficial or partial. There are no minor full thickness burns. All must be medically assessed.

Care and Management

- Call helpline immediately.
- Cool the burn for up to 20 minutes using clean cool water.
- Cover the burn with non-stick dressing.
- Treat for shock.
- Seek medical advice.

DO NOT

- Apply lotions or ointments
- Break blisters
- Apply ice directly to the burn
- Remove pieces of cloth that are stuck to the skin
- Clean burns

When cooling the face you can apply soaked towels, sheets or other wet cloths to a burned area that cannot be immersed. Ensure the material is kept wet at all times to prevent the material sticking to the skin.

The burn can be covered with moist, sterile non stick dressings to prevent infection and reduce pain. The bandage must not put pressure on the burn and the area can be elevated. If the burn covers a large area of the body, cover it with clean, moist sheets or other non-fluffy material. However it must be kept moist to prevent sticking to the skin.

If you are alone and your clothing catches fire, follow the simple guide of **"Stop, drop and roll".**

Treat scalds by removing any clothing as quickly as possible because it traps the heat. Cool the area with water and treat as for any other burn.

Chemical Burns

Cleaning solutions such as household bleach, drain cleaners, toilet bowl cleaners, paint strippers and lawn or garden chemicals often contain caustic chemicals that destroy tissues.

As long as the chemical is on the skin it will continue to burn. You must remove the chemical from the body as quickly as possible and call the ambulance. Some chemicals such as dishwasher crystals are activated by water, so brush off as much of the chemical as possible before flushing with water.

Help the casualty remove contaminated clothes and take steps to minimize shock. If an eye is burned by a chemical, keep flushing the affected eye for at least 15 minutes or until ambulance personnel arrive. Ensure that water flushes underneath the eye lids.

Warning: Blisters are actually burns. Do not attempt to decontaminate the skin where blisters have formed, as the agent has already been absorbed

Do not use ice for cooling the skin.

Synthetic materials such as nylon may melt and cause further injury.

In a chemically contaminated area, do not expose the wounds. Apply field dressing and then pressure dressing over wound area as needed.

Electrical Burns

Electrical burns can be more serious that they appear to be. The severity of an electrical burn depends on the type and amount of contact, the current's path through the body, and how long the contact lasted. Electrical burns are often deep and the casualty will have both an entrance and exit wound. Although these wounds may look superficial, the tissues below may be severely damaged. The casualty may also experience other injuries. Electricity can make the heart beat erratic or even stop.

Signs and Symptoms

- Unconsciousness
- Confused Behaviour
- Obvious burns on the skin surface
- Breathing difficulty
- Weak, irregular or absent pulse.
- Burns both where the current entered and where it left the body, often on the hand or foot.

Ensure the power has been turned off before approaching the casualty. Detach the casualty from the power lines by using wooden sticks or poles. You may need to wait for the emergency services to turn off power and stay at least 6-8 meters away. If you encounter casualties in a car that has come in contact with electricity, you must remain at a safe distance and yell your instructions to them ensuring they remain in the car.

Warning: High voltage electrical burns may cause temporary unconsciousness, difficulties in breathing, or difficulties with the heart [heartbeat].

Bleeding

Bleeding is the loss of blood from the vessels that make up the circulatory system. These vessels are known as arteries, veins and capillaries. There are two forms of bleeding, external and internal. External bleeding is obvious, whereas internal bleeding is more difficult to detect.

External Bleeding

Severe external bleeding occurs after a deep incision or laceration. The most serious bleeding is from an artery. This can be life threatening if the cut is large and under too much pressure to control. Minor bleeding usually stops by itself within 10 minutes when blood clots.

Signs and Symptoms

The signs of life-threatening external bleeding include:
- Blood spurting from a wound.
- Blood that fails to clot after all measures have been taken to control the bleeding.
- The casualty will also display signs of shock.

Care and Management

- Inspect the wound to ensure there are no objects embedded.
- Apply direct pressure to the wound.
- Lie the casualty down and elevate the affected area, if injuries permit.
- Ensure once applied that the bandage is not too tight and there is good.
- Circulation beyond the bandage.
- Monitor the casualty's pulse and breathing.
- Treat for shock.
- Call ambulance if necessary.
- Seek medical advice.

Note: If bleeding is not controlled by the initial pad, leave the initial pad in place and apply a second pad and bandage over the first. If bleeding continues through the second pad and bandage, replace the second pad and bandage. When major bleeding continues it may be necessary to remove the initial pad and bandage to ensure a specific bleeding point able to be controlled by direct pressure has not been missed.

Preventing the transmission of diseases

Ensure that you do not come in contact with your casualty's blood. There needs to be an effective barrier between you and the casualty like casualty's own hand, gloves or clean folded material.

Wash your hands with warm water and soap and dry them off effectively, both before and after care if possible and even if you wore gloves.

Avoid talking, coughing, sneezing and laughing over the casualty's open wound.

Steps to control bleeding

- Direct pressure
- Pad and bandage
- Elevation
- Treat for shock
- Blood coagulates for minor bleeding

Internal Bleeding

Internal bleeding occurs when there is a rupture of arteries, veins or capillaries. Capillary bleeding is seen in the form of bruising beneath the skin and is usually not considered serious. Deeper bleeding involving arteries or veins and may result in severe blood loss.

Internal bleeding often results from a traumatic incident such as a road accident in which there is every chance of heavy impact injuries. It is possible for the casualty to not show any signs of internal bleeding (this is very dangerous) but there may be significant damage to perhaps the liver and spleen as there is no bone coverage of the abdominal cavity. There may also be severe damage to the vessels if injured by penetrating or embedded objects.

Signs and Symptoms

- Pain at the sight
- Tenderness
- Rigid abdominal muscles
- Bleeding from other signs like coughing or vomiting blood
- Signs of shock
- Rapid, weak pulse
- Bleeding from other body orifices

Care and Management

- RABC
- Lie casualty down and rest comfortably
- Raise legs if injuries permit
- Keep casualty warm
- Reassure
- Continue to check pulse and breathing
- Call helpline
- Do not give anything to eat or drink

Warning: When the dressing is applied, do not put pressure on the wound or exposed internal parts, because pressure could cause further injury [vomiting, ruptured intestine, and so forth]. Therefore tie the dressing ties [tails] loosely at casualty's side, not directly over the dressing.

Crush Injuries

A crush injury occurs when a heavy object falls and crushes the casualty. The injuries are particularly serious when there is also damage to internal organs, bone fractures and severe bleeding.

Care and Management

- ABC
- Remove the crushing force immediately if safe to do so.
- If the casualty has not been trapped for longer than 1 hour DO NOT REMOVE the crushing force.
- Control any bleeding and other injuries.

- If unable to remove the object or the casualty has been trapped for the extended period, call for immediate help.

- Reassure the casualty and check for vital signs.

Amputations

When a part of the body is cut off or torn off, the first aider must ensure the severed area is cared for and transported to the hospital with the casualty.

Care and Management

- ABC

- Apply direct pressure to the affected limb, bandage and elevate

- Place the severed part in a plastic bag or other airtight container. Pack the bag/container into ice added to water. The severed part must never come in direct contact with water or ice. Send it to the hospital with the casualty.

Diabetes

The cells of the body not only require oxygen, but also require glucose to function normally. Food is broken down into sugar through the digestive process. Sugar requires a transportation link into the body cells. This link is called insulin, a hormone which is produced in the pancreas. Those people that do not produce enough or no insulin do not have the ability to transport their sugar into the cells of the body. Diabetes is an illness caused by the inability of the body to produce insulin.

There are two types of diabetes:

Type 1 – Insulin dependent occurs when the body produces little or no insulin. Most people with this type have to inject insulin into their body on a daily basis.

Type 2 – Non-insulin dependent occurs when the body produces insulin but not in sufficient quantity for the body's needs. These people generally control their diabetes with diet and tablet.

There are two types of conditions produced by diabetes:

Hyperglycemia – High blood sugar. This condition develops when the casualty has not taken their insulin. It is not commonly seen by first aiders as its onset is usually gradual and the casualty is able to take corrective measures.

Hypoglycemia – Low blood sugar. This condition is quick onset and if not treated can lead to unconsciousness or death. Should a diabetic inject too much insulin, miss a meal, develop an infection or over exercise, they can develop low blood sugar levels. This is the most common type of diabetes complication that a first aider will come up against.

Signs and Symptoms of Hypoglycemia (Low blood sugar)

- Weakness and/or light headed
- Confused and aggressive (Commonly mistaken for drunkenness)
- Pale, cold, sweaty skin.
- Levels of consciousness may deteriorate
- Casualty may develop seizures

Care and Management

- RABC
- Call "Emergency"
- Give the casualty something sweet to drink or eat.
- If the casualty becomes unconscious, check airway and breathing. If the casualty is breathing normally, place them into the recovery position and monitor their airway and breathing.
- If the casualty is not breathing normally, continue CPR until help arrives.

Warning: Never administer insulin to a casualty. If done incorrectly, it can be fatal.

Always seek medical advice.

The biggest problem first aider's encounter is deciding whether the casualty is suffering from high or low blood sugar. A good indicator is the casualty's skin color. If the sugar level is high the skin will be flushed and dry, if the sugar level is low the skin will be pale and sweaty.

Poisons, Bites and Stings

Poisons

There are 4 different ways poisons can enter the body:

- Ingested, that is a poison that is swallowed.
- Inhaled, as in breathing a poison into the lungs.
- Injected, such as a snakebite or hypodermic needle
- Absorbed, a poison, on contact with the skin is transferred into the body.

Care and Management

- Look around and gather possible clues.
- ABC.
- Care for life threatening conditions.
- Ask questions to gather additional information.
- Look for containers and take them with you to the telephone.
- Call helpline.

NOTE: Do not give the casualty anything to drink unless instructed to do so.

Bites and Stings

A pressure immobilization bandage is required if the casualty is bitten or stung by any of the creatures in the second section of the box given. The pressure bandage is used to slow down the transportation of the venom from the lymphatic system.

To apply the bandage:

- Apply a crepe bandage directly over the bite site to maintain pressure
- For a bite on the arm or leg, apply a second bandage and work upwards to cover as much of the limb as possible.
- Immobilize the limb to a splint or use the body as a splint
- Keep the casualty still and calm and wait for medical assistance.
- Do not remove the bandages until the casualty has reached medical care, and then only if instructed to under medical supervision.
- If the bandage has been applied too tight, circulation may be cut off to the lower parts of the limb.

Warning:

When a splint is used to immobilize the arm or leg, take extreme care to ensure the splinting is done properly and does not bind. Watch it closely and adjust it if any changes in swelling occur.

If it is an open fracture and the bone is protruding from the skin. Do not attempt to push the bone back under the skin. Apply a field dressing over the wound to protect the area.

A tourniquet is only used on an arm or leg where there is a dangerous of the casualty losing his life (bleeding to death)

The tourniquet must be easily identified or easily seen.

Do not use wire or shoestring for a tourniquet band.

Signs and symptoms of Impaired Circulation

- Numbness
- Discoloration of the fingers and toes and the sensation of coldness.

If any of these occur, loosen the bandage only enough to get circulation going in the limb again. Obviously do not attempt to use pressure immobilization technique for bites located on the head or trunk.

Ice packs – Bee, Wasp, Red Back, Scorpion, Centipede, Ants.

Pressure Bandage – Snakes, Funnel-web, Cone Shell, Blue-Ringed Octopus, Allergies.

Hot water – Stone fish, Bull trout, Stingray, Blue Bottle.

Vinegar – Box jellyfish.

Anaphylaxis

This is a term used to describe a severe allergic reaction to a substance. It is a form of shock. When a casualty comes in contact with a substance they are sensitive to, the casualty could develop anaphylaxis.

Signs and Symptoms

- Swelling at the site
- Itching or rash
- Nausea and vomiting
- Breathing difficulties may develop caused by swelling of the throat. In severe cases this could lead to an obstructed airway.

Care and Management

- ABC

- If unconscious. Lateral position and continually observe the ABC and be prepared to commence EAR/CPR as required.

- If conscious, observe the casualty and seek medical assistance.

- If the casualty has any medication for the condition, it should be taken immediately.

Warning: Insect bites/stings may cause anaphylactic shock [a shock caused by a severe allergic reaction]. This is a life-threatening event and a true medical emergency. Be prepared to perform the basic life support measures and to immediately transport the casualty to a nearest PHC/hospital.

Do not attempt to cut the bite nor suck out the venom. If the venom should seep through any damaged or lacerated tissues in your mouth, you could immediately lose consciousness or even die.

A tourniquet [a tight bandage to stop the circulation of poison] is only used on an arm or leg where there is a danger of the casualty losing his life [bleeding to death].

The tourniquet must be easily identified or easily seen.

Sprains, Strains and Fractures

Soft Tissue Injuries

Sprains involve injury to the ligaments and surrounding soft tissues

Strains involve injury to the muscles and tendons.

If in doubt as to whether the casualty has a sprain, strain, fracture or dislocation – always treat the injury as a fracture and never apply a compression bandage over a suspected broken bone.

Care and Management

The best way to remember the management of fractures is with the mnemonic RICE.

- REST – Decreases the pain.
- ICE – This applied to the injury for no longer than 10 minutes at a time. Ensure there is a barrier between the ice and the skin. Ice helps to control the swelling and relieve pain.
- COMPRESSION – A firm supportive figure 8 bandages is used to give even pressure over the injured area.
- ELEVATION – This reduces swelling as it slows the bleeding.

Fractures

The term fracture is used to describe a break in the continuity of a bone. The fracture could resemble a crack, a chip or a complete break of the bone. There are also different types of fractures:

- open fracture
- closed fracture
- complicated fracture

Warning: If an elbow fracture is suspected. Do not bend the elbow, bandage it in the position found.

If a fracture of the kneecap is suspected, do not bend the knee; bandage it in the position found.

In an open fracture, the skin around the bone is broken and the bone may be protruding. There is great risk of infection with this fracture.

In a closed fracture, the bone has broken under the skin. There may also be considerable bleeding under the skin and possible damage to muscles, vessels and soft tissues.

You suspect a casualty to have suffered a complicated fracture when there is another associated injury along with the fracture. The damage may include nerve, blood vessels or vital organs, for example when a casualty has a broken rib it may puncture the lung and that is a complication of the fracture.

Signs and Symptoms

- Pain at the site of the injury
- Swelling
- Tenderness
- Loss of movement or feeling

- Deformity
- Shock.

Care and Management

- RABC
- Control external bleeding and protect the wound.
- Ask the casualty not to move, make them comfortable.
- Avoid twisting of the neck or spine; maintain the alignment of the spine.
- Check for circulation into the limb beyond the fracture.
- Handle gently, Do Not attempt to straighten fractured limbs.
- Immobilize the fracture with pillows and blankets or use splints if necessary.
- Seek medical assistance for transportation of the casualty.
- Manage shock.

Warning: Leg fracture must be splinted before elevating the legs as a first aid measure for shock.

If a broken back or neck is suspected, do not move the casualty unless his life is in immediate danger [such as close to a burning vehicle]. Movement may cause permanent paralysis or death. When a splint is used to immobilize the arm or leg, take extreme care to ensure the splinting is done properly and does not bind. Watch it closely and adjust it if any changes in swelling occur.

Casualties with fractures of the extremities may show impaired circulation, such as numbness, tingling, cold or pale to bluish skin tone. These casualties should be evacuated by medical personnel and treated as soon as possible. Prompt medical treatment may prevent possible loss of the limb.

Do not encourage the casualty to move the injured part in order to identify a fracture since such movement could cause further damage to surrounding tissues and promote shock. If you are not sure whether a bone is fractured, care for the injury as a fracture. At the site of the fracture, the bone ends are sharp and could cause vessel [artery or vein] damage.

If it is an open fracture and the bone is protruding from the skin. Do not attempt to push the bone back under the skin. Apply a field dressing over the wound to protect the area.

Facial and Minor Wounds

Eye Injuries

The eye is very easily injured so it is therefore important that we take care when dealing with injuries to the eyes. Injuries that penetrate the eyeball or cause the eye to be removed from its socket are very serious and can cause blindness. Eye injuries can be caused in a number of ways: fists, objects, chemicals, smoke, dirt, metals.

When someone sustains an eye injury, the body tries to rectify the problem itself by creating tears to flood the object from the eye. You may also assist here by flushing the eye with water with the affected eye downwards. Do not persist in attempting to rid the eye of the object if it is stubborn. Sometimes further action needs to be taken.

Care and Management

- Call ambulance
- Rest the casualty in a comfortable position.
- Ask the casualty to close both eyes.
- Bandage only the affected eye.

- Never remove an object that is embedded in the eye. Apply padding around the object and keep the casualty still with the good eye closed until help arrives.
- Reassure the casualty.

Warning: Do not apply pressure when there is a possible laceration of the eyeball. The eyeball contains fluid. Pressure applied over the eye will force the fluid out, resulting in permanent injury. Apply protective dressing without added pressure.

Ear Wounds

Ear injuries are common and can include either outer injuries such as lacerations or inner injuries. An avulsion of the ear may occur.

When a pierced earring catches on something and tears away from the ear. To control the bleeding with an outer injury apply direct pressure to the affected area. Blood or other fluid may be in the ear canal or be draining from the ear if your casualty has sustained a head injury. As discussed earlier, do not attempt to stop this drainage but prevent infection by placing a piece of padding over the affected ear. The eardrum may be ruptured if the casualty receives a blow to the head, or perhaps an object being forced into the ear canal. Changes in the atmospheric pressure, an explosion or a deep dive can also cause injury.

If you can easily see that an insect has lodged in the ear canal you can attempt to remove it by placing a couple of drops of oil into the canal and maybe the bug will float to the top. If unsuccessful, seek medical attention.

Signs and Symptoms

- Pain
- Deafness or impaired hearing.

- Bleeding from the ear.
- Signs related to injury within the skull: watery fluid mixed with blood from the ear.
- Headache or an altered conscious state.

Care and Management

- Call ambulance.
- Position casualty comfortably, sitting up with the head tilted towards the side of the injury.
- Cover any external injuries.
- Treat for shock.

Nose Wounds

Nose injuries are usually the result of a blow to the nose and cause it to bleed. Bleeds can also be associated with high blood pressure or changes in the altitude.

Care and Management

Seat the casualty down with the head slightly forward. Ask the casualty to apply finger and thumb pressure to the soft part of the nostril for 10 minutes. Instruct the casualty to breathe through their mouth. Release the nostril after 10 minutes. If bleeding has stopped instruct the casualty not to blow or pick their nose. If bleeding is not controlled, finger and thumb pressure can continue for up to 30 minutes. If unsuccessful after the amount of time, seek medical assistance.

Warning: Do not attempt to remove objects inhaled into the nose. An untrained person who tries to remove such an object could worsen the casualty's condition and may cause permanent injury.

Do not give causalities with abdominal wounds food or water [moistening the lips is allowed].

Teeth and Mouth Wounds

If you are attending a casualty who has a tooth knocked out (to be replaced).

Care and Management

- Place the tooth in the base of the casualty's mouth and ask them to swish saliva around the tooth to clean it, or alternatively clean the tooth with milk.

- Put the tooth back into the socket and guard the tooth with a gauze pad to ensure it remains in place. Roll up some gauze and have the casualty bite down onto the gauze.

- Take the casualty to the dentist within 1 hour.

- If the tooth is to be replaced into the socket, the tooth can be transported in milk and the socket guarded with a piece of gauze.

Over Exposure to Heat

Causes

Factors affecting heat and cold related illness are:

- Humidity
- Wind
- Clothing
- Living conditions
- Work environment
- Age
- Physical activity
- Individual's health
- Over exposure to heat includes:
- Heat exhaustion/heat stress
- Heat stroke.

The most common cause of heat related illness are exercising strenuously for long periods of time and working in the hot environment. This causes the casualty to lose fluid through sweating which in turn reduces the amount of water in the body and causes the blood volume to fall. Increases blood flow to the skin to cool the casualty, further reduces blood flow and the vital organs are affected.

Signs and symptoms

- Cool, moist, pale skin
- Normal or below normal skin temperature
- Rapid, weak pulse
- Sweating
- Headache
- Nausea
- Weakness
- Dizziness.

Care and Management

- Rest the casualty lying down in a shaded area with the legs elevated
- Loosen any tight clothing
- Give small amounts of clear, cool fluids
- Sponge the skin with cool water
- It is necessary to seek medical assistance if the casualty does not recover or vomits and is unable to keep fluids down.

Heat Stroke

This is a condition described when the body's systems cease to function because the body is unable to cool itself due to the low levels of fluid. This causes the temperature to rise rapidly and can lead to convulsions, unconsciousness and death.

Signs and Symptoms

- High body temperature
- Red, hot, dry skin

- Deteriorating conscious state
- Strong pulse initially progressing to weak and irregular pulse as the blood volume drops.

Care and Management

- Rest the casualty lying down in a shaded area.
- Cool the body with cool water or ice packs in the areas of the body where the pulses can be felt, remember the 10 minute rule.
- Give cool, clear fluids only when fully conscious.
- Seek urgent medical assistance.
- If you suspect that someone has a heat stroke, immediately call emergency or transport the person to a hospital. Any delay seeking medical help can be fatal.
- While waiting for the paramedics to arrive, initiate HYPERLINK "https://www.webmd.com/a-to-z-guides/wound-care-10/slideshow-first-aid-essentials"first aid. Move the person to an air-conditioned environment -- or at least a cool, shady area -- and remove any unnecessary clothing.
- If possible, take the person's core body temperature and initiate first aid to cool it to 101 to 102 degrees Fahrenheit. (If no thermometers are available, don't hesitate to initiate first aid.)

Try these cooling techniques:

- Fan air over the patient while wetting their HYPERLINK "https://www.webmd.com/skin-problems-and-treatments/picture-of-the-skin" skin with water from a sponge or garden hose.
- Apply ice packs to the patient's armpits, groin, neck, and back. Because these areas are rich with HYPERLINK "https://www.webmd.com/heart/anatomy-picture-of-blood" blood vessels close to the skin, cooling them may reduce body temperature.

- Immerse the patient in a shower or tub of cool water.

- If the person is young and healthy and suffered heat stroke while HYPERLINK "https://www.webmd.com/fitness-exercise/default.htm" exercising vigorously -- what's known as exertional heat stroke -- you can use an ice bath to help cool the body.

- Do not use ice for older patients, young children, patients with chronic illness, or anyone whose heat stroke occurred without vigorous HYPERLINK "https://www.webmd.com/fitness-exercise/ss/slideshow-7-most-effective-exercises" exercise. Doing so can be dangerous.

Warning: the casualty should be continually monitored for development of conditions which may require the performance of necessary basic life saving measures.

Frostbite

Frostbite happens when part of the skin and other tissues freeze due to low temperatures. It can lead to loss of sensation and eventually tissue death and gangrene. This usually happens when exposed to freezing cold temperatures and windy weather.

Signs and Symptoms

- Paleness of the area and Numbness
- Hardened and stiffened Skin

Color change to the skin. The skin may change from white to mottled and blue. On recovery, the skin may be red, hot, painful and blistered. When gangrene occurs, the skin may become black due to the loss of blood supply.

Care and Management

- Help move the casualty indoors or to somewhere warm.
- Once inside, gently remove any constricting rings, gloves, boots or any other constricting items.
- Warm the affected part with your hands, in your lap.
- Do not rub the area as this could damage their skin.
- Do not place the affected part of the body on to direct heat.

Place the affected part into warm but not hot water – around 40°C. Dry the area carefully and put on a light dressing, ideally a gauze bandage from your first aid kit.

Once you've done that, help them to raise the affected part to reduce swelling. If the casualty is an adult, you can suggest they take the recommended dose of paracetamol tablets. If the casualty is a child, you can give them the recommended dose of paracetamol syrup.

Do not give aspirin to anyone under the age of 16 or anyone who is known to be allergic. Take or send them to hospital.

Hypothermia

Hypothermia is a condition that occurs when someone's body temperature drops below 35°C (95°F). Normal body temperature is around 37°C (98. 6°F). Hypothermia can become life-threatening quickly, so it's important to treat someone with hypothermia straight away.

Signs and Symptoms

- Shivering, cold and pale with dry skin
- Unusually tired, confused and have irrational behavior
- Reduced level of response
- Slow and shallow breathing
- Slow and weakening pulse.

Care and Management

Treating hypothermia outdoors

- If the casualty is outside, try to get them indoors. If you are unable to get them indoors, try to take them to a sheltered place as quickly as possible, shielding the casualty from the wind.
- Remove and replace any wet clothing and make sure their head is covered.

- Do not give them your clothes – it is important for you to stay warm yourself.

Try to protect the casualty from the ground. Lay them on a thick layer of dry, insulating material such as pine branches, heather, or bracken. If possible put them in a dry sleeping bag and/or cover them with blankets. If available, wrap them in a foil survival blanket. You can use your body to shelter them and keep them warm.

Call for Emergency help.

Do not leave the casualty alone. Somebody must be with them at all times. If you are in a remote area and cannot call for emergency help, send two people to get help together.

If the casualty is fully alert, offer them warm drinks and high energy food such as chocolate.

Monitor their breathing, level of response and temperature while waiting for help to arrive.

Treating hypothermia indoors

If you are indoors, cover the casualty with layers of blankets and warm the room to about 25°C (77°F).

Do not place any direct heat such as hot water bottles or fires near a casualty as they may cause burns.

Give them something warm to drink, like soup, and/or high-energy food, like chocolate.

Do not give the casualty alcohol in an attempt to warm them, it will make hypothermia worse.

Seek medical advice. Hypothermia could be disguising a more serious illness such as a stroke, heart attack or an underactive thyroid gland.

Monitor their breathing, level of response and temperature until they recover.

Quicksand

Quicksand isn't nearly as dangerous as it looks in the movies, it is a real phenomenon. Just about any sand or silt can temporarily become quicksand if it is sufficiently saturated with water and/or subjected to vibrations, such as those that occur during an earthquake. Here's what to do if you find yourself sinking.

Avoid quicksand. Any time you are in an area of wet ground, such as along beaches, marshes, and rivers, or if you are in a place where underground springs bubble up, you might encounter quicksand. Be on the lookout for ground that appears unstable. Often, you can't detect quicksand just by looking at it. If you step on ground that ripples or shifts beneath you, step backwards quickly and smoothly: quicksand usually takes a second or two before it liquefies.

"Walk softly and carry a big stick." When hiking, especially in an area you suspect contains quicksand, carry a long, stout pole. You can use the pole to test the ground in front of you, and you can also use it to help extract yourself should you sink.

Drop everything. Because your body is less dense than quicksand, you can't fully sink unless you panic and struggle too much (which will cause the sand to further liquidify) or you're weighed down by something heavy. If you step into quicksand and you're wearing a backpack or carrying something heavy, immediately take off your backpack or drop what you're carrying. If it's possible to get out of your shoes, do so; shoes, especially those with flat, inflexible soles (many boots, for example) create suction as you try to pull them out of quicksand. If you know ahead of time that you are highly likely to encounter quicksand, change out of your boots and either go barefoot or wear shoes that you can pull your feet out of easily.

Relax. Quicksand usually isn't more than a couple feet deep, but if you do happen to come across a particularly deep spot, you could very well sink quite quickly down to your waist. Quicksand has a density of about 2 grams per milliliter. But human density is only about 1 gram per milliliter. At that level of density, sinking in quicksand is impossible. You would descend about up to your waist, but you'd go no further. If you panic you can sink further, but if you relax, your body's buoyancy will cause you to float. Relax your head and keep your head up as much as you can without being tense.

Breathe deeply. Not only will deep breathing help you remain calm, it will also make you more buoyant. Keep as much air in your lungs as possible. It is impossible to "go under" if your lungs are full of air.

Get on your back. If you sink up to your hips or higher, bend backward. The more you spread out your weight, the harder it will be to sink. Float on your back while you slowly and carefully extricate your legs. Once your legs are free you can inch yourself to safety by using your arms to slowly and smoothly propel yourself. If you are near the edge of the quicksand, you can roll to hard ground.

Take your time. If you're stuck in quicksand, frantic movements will only hurt your cause. Whatever you do, do it slowly. Slow movements will prevent you from agitating the quicksand—the vibrations caused by rapid movements can turn otherwise relatively firm ground into more quicksand. More importantly, quicksand can react unpredictably to your movements, and if you move slowly you can more easily stop an adverse reaction and, by doing so, avoid getting yourself stuck deeper. You're going to need to be patient; depending on how much quicksand is around you, it could take several minutes or even hours to slowly, methodically get yourself out.

Get plenty of rest. Other than panic, exhaustion is your worst enemy. Since it can take a long time to get yourself out of quicksand, be sure to take breaks and just float on your back if you feel your muscles getting tired. If you're in a dangerous tidal zone, however, you may be in a race against time (see warning below).

Use a stick (optional). A stick is not necessary to extricate yourself from quicksand, but it can be helpful if you have one.

- As soon as you feel your ankles sink, lay the pole on the surface of the quicksand horizontally behind you.

- Flop onto your back on top of the pole. After a minute or two, you will achieve balance in the quicksand, and you'll stop sinking.

- Work the pole towards a new position, under your hips. The pole will prevent your hips from sinking, so you can slowly pull one leg free, then the other.

- Stay flat on your back with your arms and legs fully touching the quicksand and use the pole as a guide. Inch sideways along the pole to firm ground.

Tips

- There are a couple approaches to extricating your legs from quicksand. If the quicksand is very thick, you can move your legs in a circular motion. This will help introduce more water into the quicksand, which will make it easier to pull your legs out. You can get out using this technique, if you do it slowly and progressively. If the quicksand is not particularly thick, you should just be able to pull your legs out slowly, one at a time, as you float on your back.

- If you try one of these methods and find yourself starting to sink, stop immediately and remain calm. Breathe deeply and let yourself rest and float before trying the other method.

- If you hike with someone else in an area where you're likely to encounter quicksand, bring along at least 20 feet of rope. That way if one person falls in, the other can stand safely on firm ground and pull him out. If the person on firm ground is not strong enough to pull the victim out, the rope should be tied to a tree or other stationary object so that the victim can pull themselves out.

Warning:

- While it's possible to die of exposure (hypothermia) from being stuck in cold quicksand for an extended period of time, most quicksand-related deaths result from drowning. Most people who drown because of quicksand do so on beaches or tidal flats, where quicksand is common and where a person can become trapped as the high tide comes in. If this is a concern try to get out as quickly as possible, but still do not panic, as that will only hurt your efforts. Keep your head as high above ground (and water) as possible in order to give you more time if you are still stuck as water approaches.

- While choosing to hike barefoot may protect you from quicksand, it can expose you to parasites that enter through the skin, such as hookworms and strongholds.

- Don't ask your friends to tug on you; they're likely to pull you into two pieces if they try too hard to pull you out.

Lightning

Lightning is a big charge of electricity that can reach from clouds to the ground. There are thousands of lightning strikes every day. Scientists think that lightning hits somewhere on the earth about 100 times every second. More people are killed by lightning than by any other kind of storm, including hurricanes and tornadoes.

In the whole world, lightning kills more than 1,000 people in a year, maybe many more. A lot more people are hurt by lightning than are killed by it and many of those who live are hurt very badly. Lightning knocks many people to the ground, some are burned and some people are unconscious after they are struck.

Lightning can strike almost anywhere. Many do not understand that people can be struck before and after a rain. Lightning can strike as far as 10 miles away from a storm and 15 or more miles away from a cloud. So, if there is blue sky above you and it is not raining, you still might not be safe if you can see or hear a storm in the distance.

There is also what is called "dry lightning." That is when lightning strikes from a cloud that is not making rain. Dry lightning often causes forest fires because there is no rain to stop a fire from spreading.

Causes

Lightning strikes injure humans in several different ways:

- Direct strike, which is usually fatal.
- Contact injury, when the person was touching an object that was struck
- Side splash, when current jumped from a nearby object to the victim
- Ground strike, when current passing from a strike through the ground into a nearby victim. A strike can cause a difference of potential in the ground (due to resistance to current in the Earth), amounting to several thousand volts per foot.
- Blast injuries, either hearing damage or blunt trauma by being thrown to the ground.

Lightning strikes can produce severe injuries, and have a mortality rate of between 10 and 30%, with up to 80% of survivors sustaining long-term injuries. These severe injuries are not usually caused by thermal burns, since the current is too brief to greatly heat up tissues, instead nerves and muscles may be directly damaged by the high voltage producing holes in their cell membranes, a process called electroporation.

Care and Management

- The casualty does not carry an electrical charge and can be safely handled to apply first aid.
- Call Emergency.
- Treat for shock.
- Lightning can affect the brainstem, which controls breathing. If a victim appears lifeless, it is important to begin artificial resuscitation (CPR) immediately to prevent death by suffocation or AED if necessary.

- Transfer the patient to the nearest hospital for immediate medical attention.

Lightning Kills, Play it safe!

Facts

- No place outside is safe during a thunderstorm.
- Lightning kills more people annually than tornadoes or hurricanes.
- If you hear thunder, you are likely within striking distance of the storm. Lightning often precedes rain, so don't wait for the rain to begin before suspending activities.

Outdoors

- Plan outdoor activities to avoid thunderstorms.
- Monitor weather conditions. If you hear thunder, get inside a substantial building immediately.
- If a substantial building is not available, get inside a hard topped metal vehicle. Vehicles are safe shelter from lightning.
- Get into Lightning shelters

When none of the above are available, seek

- Dense woods
- Low lying areas
- Put feet together and Crouch. Don't let the head touch the ground. Place hands over ears to minimize hearing damage from thunder. Avoid proximity, to other people maintain a minimum of 15 ft.

Avoid

- Open areas and stay away from isolated tall objects.
- Standing or running Water
- Tall trees. Trees attract lightning.

- Metal fences
- Overhead wires and power lines
- Elevated ground
- Golf carts
- Mowers
- Cellular phones
- Radios
- Swimming

Indoor Safety

- Stay indoors and away from doors and windows.
- Unplug all valuable electronic devices. Do not use wired devices, corded phones. Lightning may strike exterior electric and phone lines, inducing shocks to inside equipment.
- Avoid contact with any equipment connected to electrical power, such as computers or appliances.
- Avoid contact with water or plumbing. No bathing or washing dishes/clothes.
- Remain inside and suspend all activities for 30 minutes after the last rumble of thunder is heard.
- Once you are in a safe place, you can take your mind off the storm by playing games, singing songs, telling stories, reading books, or doing your homework.

Warning: You can tell how far away lightning struck by counting seconds between the flash and the thunder. Every 5 seconds equals one mile, so if you count 10 seconds until you hear the thunder, the lightning flash was 2 miles away.

Sometimes you can feel when lightning might be about to strike. Try holding your arm very close to the front of a color TV screen that is turned on and see how it feels. Look at the hair standing up on your arm. If you are in or near a storm and you feel this way, then you know that you may be in danger. Lightning could strike any second.

Drowning

While near water such as pools, lakes or seaside do not force, pull or push anyone who doesn't know swimming into the water. In a near-drowning emergency, the sooner the rescue and first aid begin, the greater the victim's chance of survival.
Rescue options to reach the drowning victim

- Use a long stick, cut out a thick creeper or break off a branch.
- Throw a rope with a buoyant object, such as a life jacket.
- Bring a canoe alongside the victim and tow the victim to shore. Do not haul the victim into the boat because it may cause the boat to capsize, and both of you will be in the water. Cold water may render the victim too hypothermic to grasp objects within their reach or to hold while being pulled to safety.
- As a last resort, you can attempt a swimming rescue if you are sufficiently trained in water rescue. Do not attempt a rescue beyond your capabilities. Do not endanger yourself during this process.
- For a swimming rescue, approach the person from behind while trying to calm the victim as you move closer. A panicked victim can pull you down.
- Grab a piece of clothing or cup a hand or arm under the victim's chin and pull the person face up to shore while providing special

care to ensure a straight head-neck-back alignment especially if you think the person has spine injuries.

- The best option would be to float the victim on a board while towing to shore.

Rescue options for someone who has fallen through ice

- Do not walk on the ice to rescue someone.
- Instead, throw a rope or offer a long stick to pull the victim out and across on the ice onto the person's belly to distribute the weight as evenly as possible.
- Avoid having the victim try to climb on the ice edge because it results in more ice breaking.
- If the victim is unconscious, tie a rope around your waist, secure the other end, and slide out on the ice on your belly to reach the victim.
- Another technique is to form a human chain with everyone lying down to reach the victim.

Care and Management

- The focus of the first aid for a near-drowning victim in the water is to get oxygen into the lungs without aggravating any suspected neck injury.
- If the victim's breathing has stopped, begin mouth-to-mouth rescue breathing as soon as you safely can. This could mean starting the breathing process in the water.
- Continue to breathe for the person every five seconds while moving the victim to the shore.
- If water is swallowed making breathing difficult, perform the Heimlich maneuver (It is described in the chapter CHOKING) to clear it by hugging the victim from behind with your arms

around the victim's stomach and using the thumb side of a closed fist with your other hand on top of the fist to pull in and up. Continue these thrusts until the swallowed water is thrown out.

- Chest compressions in the water are difficult to do without a flat surface that does not give way and are reserved until such a surface is available.

- Once on shore, reassess the victim's breathing and circulation (heartbeat and pulse). If there is breathing and circulation without suspected spine injury, place the person in recovery position (lying on the stomach, arms extended at the shoulder level and bent, head on the side with the leg on the same side drawn up at a right angle to the torso) to keep the airway clear and to allow the swallowed water to drain. If there is no breathing, begin CPR. Continue CPR (chest compressions and mouth-to-mouth breathing) until help arrives or the person revives.

- Keep the person warm by removing wet clothing and covering with warm blankets to prevent hypothermia.

Remain with the recovering person until emergency medical personnel arrive.

Snake Bite

Snakebite is an injury caused by a bite from a snake. It can be dangerous and life threatening if the snake will venomous. India is the top country having the highest no. of death due to snake bite. Some specific venomous snake is responsible for this death. Till now people are not serious about that. Most of the people don't know just the first aid of snake bite. After a snake bite most village people are going to unqualified person and quacks for treatment not to hospital, this is one of the most serious causes of death. People should be aware about the sign and symptoms of snake bite and at least the first aid treatment of snakebite. In this type of emergency, victim should be admitted to nearest hospital and Anti Snake Venom (ASV) is very much necessary to save the patient life.

Venomous animals account for a large number of deaths and serious injuries all over the world. Snakes alone are estimated to inflict 2.5 million venomous bites each year, which resulting in about 125,000 deaths. But the actual number may be larger. Southeast Asia, India, Brazil, and areas of Africa have the history of large no of deaths due to only snakebite.

There are 270 species of snakes in India out of which about 60 are highly venomous. The big four dangerous snakes of India includes Indian cobra, Krait, Russell's viper and Saw-scaled viper. Almost 20000 people die due to venomous snake bites every year in India.

India is estimated to have the highest snakebite mortality in the world. World Health Organization (WHO) estimates place the number of bites to be 83,000 per annum with 11,000 deaths.

Most of the fatalities are due to the victim not reaching the hospital in time where definite treatment can be administered. In addition community is also not well informed about the occupational risks and simple measures which can prevent the bite. It continues to adopt harmful first aid practices such as tourniquets, cutting and suction, etc. Studies reveal that primary care doctors do not treat snakebite patients mainly due to lack of confidence.

Poisonous Snakes of the World

Of the more than 600 species of venomous snakes found on Earth, only about 200 can do any real damage to humans, according to the World Health Organization. The deadliest snakes on the planet are:

- Saw-Scaled Viper

    This viper, Echiscarinatus, which inhabits parts of India and the Middle East, doesn't possess the strongest of venoms, but is responsible for more human deaths annually than any other snake, partly because it's often found in populated areas.

- King Cobra

    Wondering which snake can bring down an elephant? The king cobra (Ophiophagushannah) delivers enough neurotoxins to kill an Asian elephant, as well as about 50 percent of the humans it bites. Reaching 18 feet (5.5 meters) in length, the king cobra is also the world's longest venomous snake.

- Tiger Snake

    This deadly snake (Notechisscutatus) inhabits southern Australia and Tasmania, and kills victims with a potent mixture of neurotoxins, coagulants, hemolysins and myotoxins.

Interestingly, these snakes vary greatly in size depending on their preferred type of prey.

- Inland Taipan

This reptile (Oxyuranusmicrolepidotus) is often referred to as the "fierce snake," and its bite can kill a human being in less than an hour. One of the deadliest snakes on the planet, its paralyzing venom causes hemorrhaging in blood vessels and muscle tissues.

- Faint-Banded Sea Snake

Many believe this water snake to be the most venomous snake in the world. The bite of Hydrophisbelcheri is said to be 100 times more deadly than that of its compatriot, the inland taipan. Luckily, this Indian and Pacific Ocean native is rarely known to bite humans.

- Black Mamba

The fastest snake in the world is also one of the deadliest. The black mamba (Dendroaspispolylepis) can move at speeds of up to 12.5 miles per hour (5.5 meters per second), and its bite can kill a human being in less than 30 minutes. This snake is known for using its lethal fangs to repeatedly stab those unfortunate enough to get in its way, with each bite injecting a deadly amount of neurotoxic venom.

- Indian Cobra

Indian cobra also known as "Nag". It is one of the highly venomous snakes found throughout India. Indian cobras are found in many habitats but generally in open forest edges, fields, and the areas around villages.

- Indian Krait

Krait is most dangerous venomous snake of India and one of the deadliest snakes of the world. Krait venom is extremely neurotoxic and induces muscle paralysis, its bite is lethal to man. There are 12 Species and 5 sub-species of Krait Snakes.

- Russell's Viper

  It is also called as koriwala. It is also one of the most venomous snakes all over the India. One of the most dangerous snakes of India, with an average length of 20 cm (4 ft). The dark brown or brownish-gray deadly snake feeds on Rodents, lizards & small birds.

- Indian Pit Viper

  The Indian Pit Viper is generally green in colour and also known as bamboo snake. It mainly lives on arboreal, living in vines, bushes and bamboos. They also have a very 'cool' heat sensing system.

The best solution to save people in this situation of snake bite emergency is to educate people – disseminate information about snakes and snakebite – what are snakes, when and why do they bite, how to avoid getting bitten, what to do when bitten, etc. It helps to understand that:

a. All snakes are not venomous – Every snakebite is not going to result in death.

b. Even a venomous bite is not always fatal – because the severity of snakebite depends on many factors like the size of the snake, whether the bite could be completed, whether it was a dry bite or not.

c. First Aid would enable a person to buy more time to reach medical aid on time.

d. The only cure which is available is anti-venom serum injection.

Signs and Symptoms

- Fang marks
- Severe pain

- Swelling
- Severe pain at the site
- Bleeding from wound
- Burning
- Diarrhea
- Excessive Sweating
- Blurred Vision
- Numbness/Tingling sensation
- Increased Thirst
- Nausea and vomiting
- Fever
- Loss of muscle co-ordinations
- Convulsions
- Rapid pulse
- Weakness/Dizziness/Fainting

Care and Management

- Wash wound with soap/water
- Immobilize the affected area
- Keep area slightly elevated
- Apply cool compress/wet cloth to affected part
- Apply a firm bandage 2–4 inches above bite to
    i. Prevent venom from spreading
    ii. Take care of any bleeding

- Monitor for pulse, respiration and blood pressure.
- Seek medical help as soon as possible.

Do's and don'ts

- Get the victim away from the snake
- Check the snake bite for puncture wounds. If one or two fang markings are visible, the bite is from a poisonous pit viper.
- Remember what the snake looks like. The doctor will need to know this to provide the proper treatment.
- Keep the victim calm, lying down, and with the bitten arm or leg below the level of his heart to slow the blood flowing from the wound to the heart.
- Clean the wound. Be sure to wipe away from the bite. This keeps any venom on the unbroken skin around the bite from being wiped into the wound.
- Watch for general symptom i.e. sharp pain, bruising, swelling around the bite, weakness, shortness of breath, blurred vision, and drowsiness or vomiting.
- Get the victim to the hospital as soon as possible.
- If any of the above mentioned symptoms occur within 30 minutes from the time of the bite and you are over two hours away from medical help, tie a constricting band (¾ to 1½ inches wide) two inches above the bite or above the swelling. The band needs to be loose enough to slip a finger underneath it. The band slows blood flow away from the bite, keeping the venom from reaching the heart. The band must be applied within 30 minutes after the time of the bite to be effective. If the swelling spreads, move the band so that it is two inches above the swelling.

- Protect the victim and others from further bites. While identifying the species is desirable in certain regions, risking further bites or delaying proper medical treatment by attempting to capture or kill the snake is not recommended.
- Keep the victim calm acute stress reaction increases blood flow and endangers the person. Panic is infectious and compromises judgment.
- Call for help to arrange for transport to the nearest hospital emergency room where anti venom for snakes common to the area will often be available.
- Make sure to keep the bitten limb in a functional position and below the victim's heart level so as to minimize the blood returning to the heart and other organs of the body.
- Do not give the victim anything to eat or drink. This is especially important with consumable alcohol, a known vasodilator which will speed up the absorption of venom. Do not administer stimulants or pain medications to the victim unless specifically directed to do so by a physician.
- Remove any items or clothing which may constrict the bitten limb if it swells (rings, bracelets, watches, footwear etc)
- Keep the victim as still as possible.
- Do not incise the bitten site.

Prevention

- Do not attempt to kill the snake
- If you spot a snake, leave it alone.
- While hiking or in the woods, stay out of tall grass
- Do not put your hand into pits/crevices during treks
- Exercise caution while climbing rocks

Many organizations, including the American medical association and American Red Cross recommend washing the bite with soap and water. Australian recommendations for snake bite treatment recommend against cleaning the wound. Traces of venom left on the skin/bandages from the strike can be used in combination with a snake bite identification kit to identify the species of snake. This speeds determination of which anti venom to administer in the emergency room.

India developed a national snake bite protocol in 2007 which includes advice to;

Reassure the patient. 70% of all snakebites are from non venomous species only 50% of bites by venomous species actually envenomate the patient.

Immobilize in the same way as a fractured limb. Use bandages or cloth to hold the splints not to block the blood supply or apply pressure. Do not apply any compression in the form of tight ligatures they don't work and can be dangerous.

Get to hospital immediately. Traditional remedies have no proven benefit in treating snakebite.

Tell the doctor of any systemic symptoms such as ptosis that manifest on the way to hospital.

Blood Donation

In most cases of emergency, either there is a loss of blood or a need for surgery and therefore a requirement of blood. Blood has no alternatives. Blood can't be produced artificially or chemically. Blood has to come from donors only.

Lakhs of people are in need of blood to save their lives. The demand is more than the supply. Any healthy human between the ages of 18 to 55 can donate blood. Though the normal human body has 5 litres of blood, the body requires only 3.5 litres of blood to function normally. The body therefore has an excess of 1.5 litres. Only 350 ml of blood is accepted from any person in a single donation. This amount of blood is also reproduced by the body in a maximum of three months' time. The donor's health also improves with the rush of fresh blood.

Donating blood is safe, simple and almost painless. Donating blood is a life saving measure especially when you have a rare blood type. It takes only about 10-15 minutes to donate blood - less than the time of an average telephone call. You can save up to 3 to 4 precious lives by donating blood because blood is separated into its components and given to different patients according to their need.

This is what you can expect when you are ready to donate blood:

- You walk into a reputed and safe blood donation centre or a mobile camp organized by a reputed institution.

- A few questions will be asked to determine your health status (general questions on health, donation history etc). Usually you will be asked to fill out a short form.
- Then a quick physical check will be done to check temperature, blood pressure, pulse and hemoglobin content in blood to ensure you are a healthy donor.
- If found fit to donate, then you will be asked to lie down on a resting chair or a bed. Your arm will be thoroughly cleaned. Then using sterile equipments blood will be collected in a special plastic bag.

"Let every heart pump with joy – Donate blood"

You can donate blood if your weight is 45 kgs or more, your hemoglobin is 12.5 gm% minimum and have not suffered from malaria, typhoid or other transmissible disease in the recent past.

There are many situations in which patients need blood to stay alive:

- In miscarriage or childbirth cases the patient may need large amount of blood to be transfused for saving her life and also the child's.
- For patients with blood diseases like severe Anemias especially a plastic Anemias, Leukemias (blood cancer), Hemophilia (bleeding disorder), Thalassemia etc. repeated blood transfusions are the only solution.
- In many other situations like poisoning, drug reactions, shock, burns, blood transfusion is the only way to save precious human life.
- On average, a hip replacement typically uses one unit of blood, a cardiac bypass 2units, a heart transplant 2units, open heart surgery about 6 units and a liver transplant 10units!
- Statistics show that 45 percent or more of us will require blood at least once in our lifetime.

Who knows, some day in case of emergency even if you need blood, donors have to come forward. NO OTHER WAY.

Consider Starting A Blood Donor Pool in Your Local Area/Among Friends/Organization With The Following Criteria

The members would donate and receive blood whenever there is a need only. They give their consent and the pool will avail the service when needed. Their good work is recorded with appreciation and returned with humility, in case of emergency (ICE). Assured of such an act, when they themselves or their dear ones need the most, the members will build up his points whenever they can, to avail when needed.

Process of give and take - benefit for all.

Be A Voluntary Blood Donor and Save Lives.

Get as many youngsters you know to donate blood.

Eye Donation

Do you know that our eyes can live even after our death? Do you know that we can light the life of a blind person by donating our eyes after our death? Do you know that eye donation is the noblest of all causes?

Join and Enroll in this Initiative To Enable The Blind To See and Lead a Colorful Life!-Like YOU

Lakhs of blind people are waiting to be bestowed with the god's gift of Vision/Sight!

A great gesture from YOU can give vision to TWO BLIND people! So, go ahead and act on this noble cause so that you can make some contribution to the society and the needy!

Service to humanity is service to GOD and the best work of life.

Your eyes can add light to someone's life. Let your eyes change someone's life.

Any human being from the age of 1year can be a donor without any maximum age limit for donating the eyes. The gender, blood group, race and health conditions don't interfere. All one needs to do is bequeath his or her eyes by taking a simple pledge to donate the eyes after death. While taking a pledge during one's lifetime itself is a noble deed, it requires the support of the relatives or friends to carry out the wishes of eye donation of the deceased.

- People using spectacles, suffering diabetes or hypertension and who had cataract surgery too can donate eyes. Persons blind from retinal or optic nerve disease can also donate their eyes.

- You need to call up the Eye Bank as soon as possible as the eyes are to be removed within a maximum of six hours of death.

- The blind can see this beautiful world, through your eyes! - Pledge Your Eyes, Gift Your Sight - Make it your WISH!

Please remember the following after making the call to the Eye Bank.

- Keep both eyes of the deceased closed and cover them with moist cotton.

- Switch off the ceiling fan, if any, directly over the deceased person and switch on the AC if available.

- If possible, apply antibiotic eye drops periodically in the deceased's eyes to reduce the chance of any infection.

- Raise the head of the deceased by placing a pillow, if possible, to reduce the chances of bleeding at the time of removal of the eyes.

Motivate the relative of the deceased person to donate the eyes. This worthy act of yours would go a long way in making INDIA blind-free. You are authorized to donate the eyes of your beloved relative at the time of their death, even if a pledge for donation has not been made earlier by the deceased. At the site, the eyes of the deceased are enucleated without causing any disfigurement. This procedure takes about 10–15 minutes. Eyes are collected and distributed free of cost. The donation is kept confidential.

See what your eyes can do for others-GRANT VISION.

You can cure blindness – take a minute

Don't you think it is time to pledge your eyes too?

A sincere appeal to you

- Pledge to donate your eyes.
- Motivate and educate others particularly the senior citizens about eye donation.
- In case of anybody's death; motivate the close relative of the deceased person to
- Donate the eyes.
- Call toll free 1919 to know your nearest eye bank.

I have pledged my eyes – have you?

Pledge

I_____ pledge to donate my eyes. I hereby request my family/relatives/friends to contact the nearest eye bank at the time of my death and donate my eyes. I have informed about this pledge to all my kith and kin.

Place:

Date: Signature of the donor

Please note that this pledge need not be sent anywhere for registration. It is to be kept in your house and your relatives informed about the pledge.

Earnest appeal especially to doctors, nurses, priests, close relatives: Upon the death of anyone please motivate the persons concerned to donate the eyes of the deceased. By doing so, you will be rendering a great service to humanity.

Don't burn or bury – which you can gift – Donate Eyes

Get as many senior citizens you know to pledge to donate their eyes.

Organ Donation

Lakhs of people have lost their lives when a vital organ failed to function in their body. Medical advances in the field of transplantation, surgical management and organ preservation have made the transplantation of vital organs possible. This system provides a viable approach to the management of diseases that cause irreversible organ failure and help precious lives from being lost before their time.

Organ donation means that a person during his lifetime pledges that after brain death, organs from his/her body can be transplanted to terminally ill patients to give them a new lease of life. The major donor organs and tissues are heart, lungs, liver, pancreas, kidneys, eyes, heart valves, skin, bones, bone marrow, connective tissues, middle ear, and blood vessels. Therefore, one donor can possibly give gift of life to as many as fifty individual terminally ill patients who would not survive otherwise.

Life is too precious to be lost to an organ failure.

Anyone, regardless of age, race or gender can become an organ and tissue donor and register at a reputed organ donor registry.

Organ Donation Registry, is set up with a purpose of

- Encouraging organ donations,
- Fair and equitable distribution
- Optimum utilization of human organs.

This registry maintains

- Waiting list of terminally ill patients requiring transplants, donor registration, matching of recipients with donor, co-ordination from procurement of organs to transplantation, dissemination of information to all concerned hospitals, organizations and individuals, creating awareness, promotion of organ donation and transplantation activities.

Donors, who have during their lifetime consented for organ donation in writing in the presence of two witnesses (at least one of whom is a close relative), are advised to express their wishes to their near and dear ones and also carry their donor cards,

Organ Donation Pledge	
I, do hereby make this anatomical gift, if medically acceptable, to take effect upon my brain death. I wish to donate the following organs: Kidneys Lungs Heart Liver Eyes	
Donor's Name	Address
Sex	Contact No.
Age	Special wishes
Blood Group	Signature
Witness: 1) 2)	

In case no such consent or donor pledge form was filled before death, then the next of kin are authorized to give consent for organ donation. The attending doctor will always ask the permission for organ donation from the family even though the person's signed card is sighted. Therefore, it is important that the donor discuss his/her decision with family members and loved ones so that it will be easier for them to fulfill the donor's wish.

What is brain death?

It is the irreversible and permanent cessation of all brain functions. Brain can no longer send messages to the body to perform vital functions like breathing, sensation, obeying commands etc. Such persons are kept on artificial support (ventilation) to maintain oxygenation of organs so that the organs are in healthy condition until they are removed. Most cases of brain death are the end result of head injuries, brain tumors patients from Intensive care units. Organs of such patients can be transplanted in organ failure patients to provide them a new lease of life.

A highly skilled surgical transplant team removes the organs and tissues and stitch up the body carefully, hence no disfigurement occurs. The appearance of the body is not altered. The body can be viewed as in any case of death. The removal or organs or tissues will not interfere with customary funeral or burial arrangements and they need not be delayed.

Healthy organs should be transplanted as soon as possible after brain death from the donor to the recipient. The donor's vital organs will be transplanted to those individuals who need them most urgently. Gifts of life (Organs) are matched to recipients on the basis of medical suitability, urgency of transplant, duration on the waiting list and geographical location. There is no charge or payment for such organ/tissues donations used in transplantations. Organ donation is a true gift.

PROCESS

- Hospital Organ Donation Registry (HODR) coordinates the process of cadaver organ donation i.e. organ donation after death and transplantation.
- There are two ways to donate organs:
    - By pledging for organ donation when a person is alive
    - By consent of family after death.

- During lifetime, a person can pledge for organ donation by filling up a donor form in the presence of two witnesses, one of who shall be a near relative.

- The organ donor form could be obtained from HODR either personally or through mail. It could also be downloaded from the hospital website.

- The donor form is absolutely free of cost.

- As mentioned earlier, you need to fill up the donor form and get it signed by two witnesses one of whom shall be a near relative and send the same to HODR

- After receiving the filled in form, HODR provides the donor with an organ donor card bearing registration number on it.

- It is suggested to keep the donor card in your pocket and share your decision with your near and dear ones.

- If a person expires without registration, the family members can donate his/her organs. For this they need to sign a consent form, which is provided at that time.

- Once, the relatives give a written consent, organs are harvested within a few hours.

- The family of the donor does not face any difficulty or extra burden upon them.

- The transplant coordination team carries out the entire process till the relatives receive the body of the deceased.

- The deceased body is given back to the family in a dignified way.

- There is no disfigurement. The body can be viewed as in any case of death and funeral arrangements need not be delayed.

God forbid, envision how your dear one suffering an organ failure would long wait with mixed feelings on that waiting list and long for another loved ones organ donation.

Note

- It is legal by law. The government of India has enacted the "transplantation of human organs act 1994" in Feb. 1995, which has allowed organ donation and legalized brain death.

- The organs can only be removed when a person is brain dead in the hospital and is immediately put on a ventilator and other life support systems. If it is a death at home, only eyes and tissues can be removed.

- Medical suitability for donation is determined at the time of death.

- So, all you need to know and do is pledge for donation.

Some terminal diseases which can be cured by organ transplantation

Heart – heart failure,

Lungs – terminal lung illness,

Kidneys – kidney failure,

Liver – liver failure,

Pancreas – diabetes,

Eyes – blindness,

Heart valve – Valvular disease,

Skin – severe burns

Without bone marrow, blood cannot be produced. When things go wrong and the bone marrow becomes damaged, for example as a result of treatment for leukemia or a related cancer of the blood, the patient must receive a transplant to survive.

There are two ways of Organ donation:

- *Living related donors:* only immediate blood relations (brother, sister, parents & children) can donate as per the Transplantation of Human Organ Act 1994. Living donor can donate only few organs, one kidney (as one kidney is capable of maintaining the body functions), a portion of pancreas (as half of the pancreas is adequate for sustaining pancreatic functions) and part of the liver (as the few segments that are donated will regenerate after a period of time) can be donated.

- *Cadaver Organ donor:* can donate all organs after brain death.

First Aid Training Institutes

By now you should be more than interested in taking a first aid course/CPR course. For more details on courses contact any of the recognized and reputed training institutes in your local area/the Indian Red Cross. Here is a list of training institutes to get you started if living in India.

24x7 Medical Service

Address: A-69/1, HariKoti Road, AbulFazl Enclave, Jamia Nagar, New Delhi, Delhi – 110 025, India

Phone: +(91)-(11)-64723799

Mobile/Cell Phone: +(91)-9891533071

Website: http://www.indiamart.com/24x7medicalservice/

Omega School of Industrial Management

Address: 20, Zachariah Colony, Choolaimedu, Chennai, Tamil Nadu – 600 094, India

Phone: +(91)-(44)-65435608

Website: http://www.indiamart.com/company/933302/

VasundharaEhs Management Consultancy

Address: S.No. 22, Dhanshree Building, Balajinagar, Dhankawadi Pune, Maharashtra, Pune, Maharashtra – 411043, India

Mobile/Cell Phone: +(91)-9595400405

Website: http://www.indiamart.com/company/2495995/

Knightdetectivesecurity

Address: No.15, First Floor, Tower – A, Unadeep Shopping Complex, SusenTarsali Ring Road, Vadodara, Gujarat – 390 010, India

Phone: +(91)-(265)-2634128/6545016

Website: http://www.indiamart.com/knight-detective-security/

Safety Circle National Safety Council

Address: DLF-G – 14/4 Phase I, Gurgaon, Haryana – 122 001, India

Mobile/Cell Phone: +(91)-9212738312/9717014831

Website: http://www.indiamart.com/company/2528512/

Institute of Safety

Address: 11 & 12, Upper Gr. Floor, ShubhLaxmi Complex, City Light, Opposite Bank Of Baroda, Surat, Gujarat – 395 007, India

Phone: +(91)-(261)-6458677

Mobile/Cell Phone: +(91)-9825067746

Website: http://www.indiamart.com/company/1601750/

Institute For Fire & Safety

Address: Ground Floor, Matruchhaya, Gulmohor Lane, Near IDEMI, Chunabhatti East, Mumbai, Maharashtra – 400 022, India

Phone: +(91)-(22)-24056676/26859598 **Fax:** +(91)-(22)-24056676

Mobile/Cell Phone: +(91)-9324495439

Website: http://www.indiamart.com/company/2110224/

ShatrunjayaMedisource SIMS

Address: MeghShraman Apartment, City Light, Surat, Gujarat – 395 007, India

Phone: +(91)-(261)-4023001

Mobile/Cell Phone: +(91)-9824509455

Website: http://www.indiamart.com/company/2175456/

Health First Medicorp

Address: Floor No. 04, Rathivilla, Desmukhwadi, NDA Road, Shivne, Pune, Maharashtra – 411 023, India

Phone: +(91)-(20)-32911329

Mobile/Cell Phone: +(91)-9028531976/9970505128

Website: http://www.indiamart.com/company/3034344/

SMR Health & Safety Solutions

Address: 401, Shree Shivdutta Reddy Apartments, Topiwala Lane, Near lalit Restaurant, Goregaon(West),, Mumbai, Maharashtra – 400 104, India

Phone: +(91)-(22)-28722981

Mobile/Cell Phone: +(91)-9867113070

Website: http://www.indiamart.com/company/3336672/

Rajans Vigil Security And Allied Services

Address: 214, Mahalakshmi KrupaKarumariamman Temple Street Whitefield -Post, Bangalore, Karnataka – 560066, India

Phone: +(91)-(80)-32438686/28451013 Fax: +(91)-(80)-28451013

Mobile/Cell Phone: +(91)-9845048890

Website: http://www.indiamart.com/rvsa-services/

Principal Hr

Address: Flat No: 004, Plot No: 317, MythriNilayam, UshaMullapudi Colony (Hal Colony), Opposite: Umcc, Gajularamaram Road, I D A Jeedimetla, Hyderabad, Andhra Pradesh – 500 055, India

Mobile/Cell Phone: +(91)-9848815425/9396961933

Website: http://www.indiamart.com/company/3510751/

Providence International

Address: Off 406, MG Road, Pune, Maharashtra – 411 001, India

Phone: +(91)-(20)-41282922 Fax: +(91)-(20)-41282922

Mobile/Cell Phone: +(91)-9763563067

SMR Health & Safety Solutions

Address: No. 401, Shree Shivdatta Reddy Apartments, To Lane, Goregaon, West, Mumbai, Maharashtra – 400 104, India

Phone: +(91)-(22)-28722981 Fax: +(91)-(22)-28722981

Mobile/Cell Phone: +(91)-9867113070

Arbrit Safety And Engg Solutions Private Limited

Address: Cc 35/1,439, Kochaneth Building, 1st Floor, N. H. Road, Near St. Martin Church, Palarivattom, Kochi, Kerala – 682 025, India

Phone: +(91)-(484)-6492025 Fax: +(91)-(484)-2339960

Priyanka Holistic Health Care System

Address: Flat No. G-2, KBR Residency, Pawani Estate, Bhandari Layout, Near Bhandari Ganapati Temple, Nizampet Village, Hyderabad, Andhra Pradesh – 500 090, India

Phone: +(91)-(40)-42000082

Mobile/Cell Phone: +(91)-9493406018

Indian Red Cross Society, Chandigarh

Address: Indian Red Cross Society, UT Branch, 2 Floor, KarunaSadan, Building Sector 11 B, Chandigarh, Chandigarh – 160 011, India

Phone: +(91)-(172)-2744188

Mobile/Cell Phone: +(91)-9463456747

St. John Ambulance, Chennai

Address: 721, M. T. H. Road, Mannurpet, Chennai, Tamil Nadu – 600 050, India

Phone: +(95)-(44)-26242318/32915643 **Fax:** +(95)-(44)-26242038

Mobile/Cell Phone: +(95)-9840799786

J K Occupational Health Centre Private Limited

Address: 78 - B, Shiveshish Flats, Mane Tilasta, Mujmahuda, Vadodara, Gujarat – 390 020, India

Phone: +(91)-(265)-2327737

Mobile/Cell Phone: +(91)-9825411780

St. John Ambulance Association

Address: No. 12, Vannier Street, Choolaimedu, Chennai, Tamil Nadu – 600 094, India

Mobile/Cell Phone: +(91)-9382645796

Conferences India

Address: 151, 3rd Floor, Dda Flats, ShahpurJat, New Delhi, Delhi – 110 049, India

Phone: +(91)-(11)-30892749 **Fax:** +(91)-(11)-30892629

Mobile/Cell Phone: +(91)-9818081565/9958244995

Website: http://www.indiamart.com/company/468095/

VasundharaEhs Management Consultancy

Address: S.No. 22, Dhanshree Building, Balajinagar, Dhankawadi Pune, Maharashtra, Pune – 411043, India

Mobile/Cell Phone:+(91)-9595400405

Website: http://www.indiamart.com/company/2495995/

Safety Circle National Safety Council

Address: DLF? G - 14/4 Phase I, Gurgaon – 122 001, India

Mobile/Cell Phone: +(91)-9212738312/9717014831

Website: http://www.indiamart.com/company/2528512/

Health First Medicorp

Address: Floor No. 04, Rathivilla, Desmukhwadi, NDA Road, Shivne, Pune – 411 023, India

Phone: +(91)-(20)-32911329

Mobile/Cell Phone: +(91)-9028531976/9970505128

Website: http://www.indiamart.com/company/3034344/

Institute For Fire & Safety

Address: Ground Floor, Matruchhaya, Gulmohor Lane, Near IDEMI, Chunabhatti East, Mumbai – 400 022, India

Phone: +(91)-(22)-24056676/26859598 **Fax:** +(91)-(22)-24056676

Mobile/Cell Phone: +(91)-9324495439

Website: http://www.indiamart.com/company/2110224/

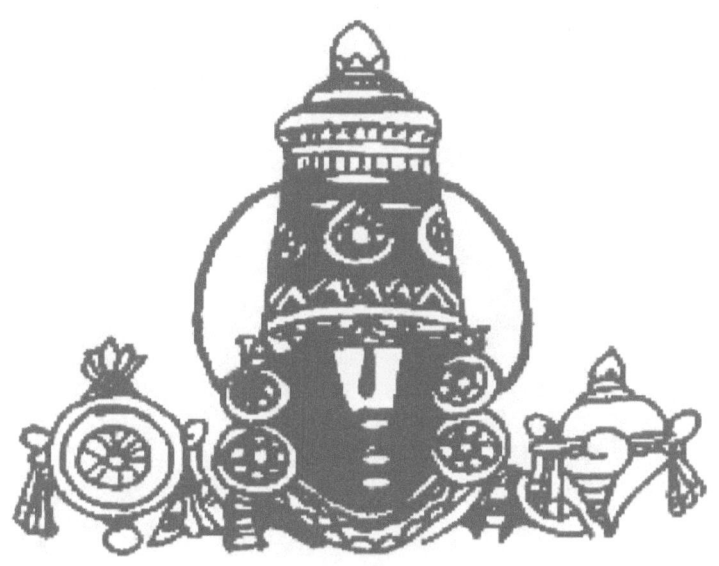

SarveJanaSukhinoBhavanthu – SamasthaSanmangalaniSanthu

May everyone be happy – May good things happen.

Om Shanthi, Shanthi, Shanthi

May peace, peace and peace alone prevail.

www.ingramcontent.com/pod-product-compliance
Lightning Source LLC
Chambersburg PA
CBHW030752180526
45163CB00003B/992